EXPLANATORY NOTE
FOR THOSE WHO DO NOT KNOW:

Erythrocytes, or red blood cells,
are the red cells.

Leukocytes, or white blood cells,
are the white cells.

**There are more people healed
by holistic treatments than
by allopathic methods.**

Table of Contents

WE ARE *NOT* WHAT WE EAT

We *ARE* What We Do Not DIGEST and ASSIMILATE!

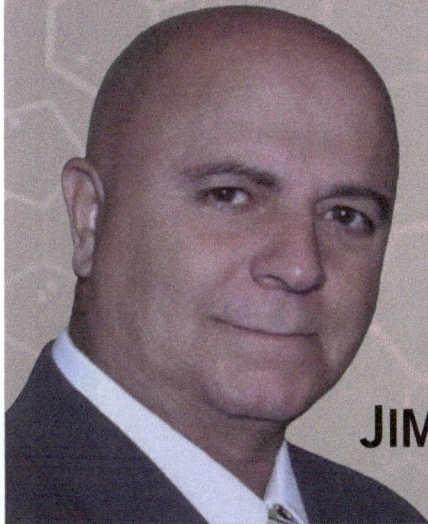

THE TRUTH ABOUT WHY OUR BODY GETS SICK

JIMMY ALBUQUERQUE

"We are not human beings! We are spiritual beings who inhabit human bodies. The body was given to us for our spiritual evolution, and it is ours to care for."

WE ARE *NOT* WHAT WE EAT

We *ARE* What We Do Not DIGEST and ASSIMILATE!

THE TRUTH WHY OUR BODY GETS SICK

BY JIMMY ALBUQUERQUE

Paperback: ISBN: 978-1-957528-06-9

Kindle-Mobi eBook: ISBN: 978-1-957528-07-6

Published by LAURUS BOOKS USA

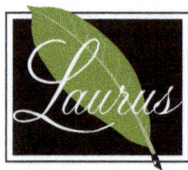

LAURUS BOOKS
THE LAURUS COMPANY, INC.
www.TheLaurusCompany.com

This book may be purchased in paperback from TheLaurusCompany.com, all Amazon affiliates, and most other retailers around the world. Available to retailers in Spring Arbor. May also be available in Kindle format for electronic readers and in audio.

Table of Contents cont.

Dr. RENATO MENEGUELO
Creator of Phosphoethanolamine

There are countless scientific articles reporting that Glioblastoma Multiforme (GBM) Level 4 has no cure, even after surgery, chemotherapy and/or radiotherapy. However, this book shows the results that Jimmy Albuquerque achieved with his blood cleaning therapy in curing his disease, in spite of it being considered incurable by the scientific community that still denies there is a cure. He became a brother and a friend while I was sick with the same histological type of cancer (GBM), considered inoperable and, as far as medicine goes, also incurable. Jimmy was first healed himself, and today brings hope to everyone in his sphere.

With him, I increased my faith and realized that God never leaves us to be alone. So, he is my brother and friend, a man with a clean heart and a clear mind in search of what many think is impossible—the cure for cancer. Worthy of the respect of everyone around him, he has one of the most brilliant minds I have had the pleasure of meeting. He has great faith in his work, his family life, and with friends. May this book bring comfort to those in need so that they know that God will always send an alternative. I myself was a man of science only, and of little faith. It was Mr. Jimmy who showed me that without faith there is no science, because research revolves around believing, and if you don't believe in your work, it is not science but a waste of time! In any case, we are cured!

Continued next page

Professor Renato Meneguelo, Neurologist, Oncologist, Neurologist with a background in Traffic Medicine, a master's degree in Bioengineering and a PhD in Medical Sciences at USP (São Paulo University-Brasil), and Fine Chemistry at ITA (Technological Institute of Aeronautics), Director of Research at Sírio Libanês hospital in Paraguay.

And Personal Friend of Dr. Jimmy Albuquerque.

ISMAEL FABREGAS

What can I say about Jimmy? What should I say about the decisive Pernambuco native who, since childhood growing up in Rio de Janeiro, already felt an imperious command inside himself. That drive convinced him to seek the TRUTH everywhere it could be available in the world and among all peoples. He lived in and traveled throughout Brazil, the United States, Europe, Africa, India, and the East, getting involved with the most heterogeneous cultures, with commoners, with aristocracy, the intellectuals, the wise, and also with the most simple peoples, led by a Universal Superior Mind, driven by boundless courage and personally undeterred. He managed to encapsulate the knowledge that he teaches today with a unique way in his language and in ways he strives to reach and help everyone.

Possessing a magnetic talent to communicate with people, an enlightened intelligence, he came to my aid when he saw me dejected, during the most turbulent moments of my life. He would always say, "There is no problem without a solution, there is no solution without defect, and there is no defect that cannot be corrected with time." Jimmy himself practices everything he has learned. When he lived in Africa, he was given the honorary title of "Master Jimmy" for the pride of his spirit, for his respect for the unprotected, for his fearlessness, for the dignity and honor with which he fought against the oppression and prejudices that reduce human value. Pages could be filled out describing Jimmy, but he is an open book for all to read. And as always, he embraces all who come to him with an affectionate embrace. The more he helps others, the more rewarded he feels. Jimmy Albuquerque certainly believes he is guided by spiritual intuition of the Divine Mind, and has an immense reservoir of great spiritual universal truths.

He clearly demonstrates today, after having overcome a mortal illness, that by divine providence and through the challenges posed to him, the blessed gratitude for offering the earthly brothers the same gift, until then very rare, that he received. Jimmy Albuquerque feels the supreme duty to share with all the brothers and sisters, the chapters of an authentic treasure, making him an able guide of the most religious traditions on our planet. With all admiration, respect, and immense appreciation.

Your friend,

Ismael Fábregas

Continued next page

Ismael Fábregas was born in Belo Horizonte MG, has over 20 years of residency and works in the United States and Europe. He is an international lawyer and holds a law degree from the Federal University of Minas Gerais, a postgraduate degree in Administrative Sciences from the University of Scientific Management of Minas Gerais, specializing in Business Administration from Fundação João Pinheiro and a postgraduate degree in International Law and Marketing Management from Columbia University, New York, NYC, USA. He is Executive and International Director of *Sister Cities Magazyne.*

Your future is determined by who you honor.

Dr. MARILENE NEVES

I am very grateful to God, who through my brother, allowed me to meet Jimmy, a man with a big heart who gave me the opportunity to experience his beautiful work in recovering the health of his patients.

Jimmy Albuquerque is a great friend, a persevering Christian who is convinced of his actions. A human being who is always willing to collaborate for a better world, seeking to bring his precious knowledge and experience to those who need a word of hope, peace, and responsibility to achieve their much-desired health. Jimmy's work is filled with patience and love and is rich in all social welfare. Jimmy Albuquerque, with whom I had the opportunity to work, deserves not only professional attention but also a contribution to the activity in my company. I am very grateful to God who allowed me, through my brother, to meet this perfect man of great and special moments. Thank you, friend, that God continues to light your way so that you can accomplish your mission.

Dr. Marilene Neves
Clinical Psychologist Responsible for ESALT -
Espaço Alternativo Saúde - Brasília / DF

We are made of the same material that dreams are made of.
                                                    —Shakespeare

PAULO ABREU

I have known Jimmy Albuquerque for many years, and my earliest memory of our first meeting was right at the beginning of my arrival in the U.S. back in 2001, when I entered his real estate company in Pompano Beach, to negotiate real estate deals. Since then, we have occasionally met at events and venues in the Brazilian community. I once heard comments that his wife had been diagnosed with cancer, and he was doing everything to help her recover in the process.

Unfortunately, in this fight, who became champion was the disease, and his wife sadly passed away. Jimmy suffered a deep loss. Some time passed, and the news came to me that it was now his turn to wrestle with this disease. One day, walking into a restaurant, I ran into Jimmy, and I was terrified because he was not the same person I had met before.

He was transformed by the disease and the chemotherapy treatments, very thin (cadaverous was more like it), with a sad look and already being overcome by the disease. I was saddened by the condition of my friend and already prepared myself for the potential loss, as it seemed irreversible to him. Months went by, and I heard no more about him until, one day, a personal friend, a dear pastor, who was struggling with cancer in his wife, presented at a meeting of Pastors who thanked everyone for their prayers and said: *Thank God for the healing of my wife, and my friend Jimmy who was the instrument of God to heal her.*

I was shocked. After the meeting, I looked for my friend and went to see if it was the same Jimmy. And what was my surprise? Jimmy had been cured of cancer in California and was now helping people to treat themselves and cleanse their blood. I was doubly happy.

As a Life Coach, I need to maintain my health at a high level, so I went to visit him at his home, and I did my blood test to check my health, and from then on, I started referring my family and friends to be treated by him. I usually say that any professional can do this type of live blood test and give the diagnoses of what the microscope shows, but the way Jimmy treats this subject is totally different. He has tremendous respect for people, a real passion for life, and great love for his patients, dedicating only to God the Lordship over human life. When he decided to take the LIFE COACH course at our Institute, I asked: "What motivates you to pursue this type of course with us?" His response was even more surprising. He told me: "Paulo, I really want to help my patients to heal from these diseases, and I want to learn all the techniques and tools that everyone has for self-help, so that I can motivate my patients to do the treatment and remain firm until they are cured, and I'll learn all the self-help techniques and tools to motivate my patients to get treatment and stay firm until healed. I don't want them to sabotage themselves in the process and lose their lives. I want to be the inspiration and motivation for them, and coaching will give me these tools." With this big

Continued next page

loving heart, deep dedication to his patients, with a great deal of personal and family sacrifice due to the extensive trips, Jimmy has become this great beacon and professional in this fight against cancer.

HE IS DETERMINED TO WIN THE WAR AGAINST CANCER.

May you have great success in your fight against disease, with favor from GOD.

Pastor Paulo Abreu
Master Trainer Coach

Endorsements

PASTOR JOSE ROBERTO FRESCHI DE OLIVEIRA

I met Jimmy Albuquerque in 2012 via cousins who live in Miami who sought him for a cure of a serious illness. Sometime after we initially met, they were physically restored. Since 2012, I have accompanied Jimmy on his visits to São Paulo. He lives for a unique purpose, to bring hope, faith, joy, determination, purpose, and disposition to people, many of them hopeless through sickness. I am an eyewitness to some amazing results. Jimmy went through the worst, or one of the worst, types of cancer, where medicine says there is no cure, Glioblastoma Multiforme (GBM). He "decided" to cure himself, and today he is a living witness to the Ministry he exercises. He is a great friend and brother that I am honored to have. If someone needs advice, or spiritual comfort, or an alternative to healing, I advise you to read this book and understand the few things we must know. Jimmy's approach is totally different from what we think in life. Jimmy embodies what we really need to know in this area of health.

José Roberto Freschi de Oliveira
Business Administrator,
Coach (CIS - Integral Systemic Coaching),
Morphologist by ABA,
American Blood Analysis Corp., and
evangelical pastor.

Acknowledgements

*B*efore we go any farther in this book, I want to thank God immensely, as well as the people who urged me to write this book:

- I dedicate this book to my children: Stanley, Jennifer, and Phillip, who have always been my beloved and most dedicated supporters.

- I would also like to express my appreciation for those who obtained a cure for sicknesses ranging from minor illnesses to those who were terminally ill who obtained healing by believing in and adhering to the therapeutic guidelines presented in this book.

- Finally, I want to thank you, the reader, in that through reading this book, you will have an excellent resource for your physical and mental well-being. As well, we pray that you will forward the information contained herein to anyone in need.

Introduction

This book will give you a better understanding of HEALTH and practical instruction. I have lived numerous life experiences in this lifetime, having gone through many different moments of joy, gains, losses, sadness, and personal fulfillment. My recent experience of developing a cure for Glioblastoma Multiforme Level 4 is the basis for this book, and also from those people who followed my therapy and got healed. Until recently, this type of brain cancer had been considered incurable. Please use this knowledge as a primer to keep your health or to self-heal from any disease. What I have written here is partly experience coupled with lessons learned, acquired from a lifetime of reading, learning, and imitating the essentials that I came to terms with in my life.

"If you are an Eagle, don't join the chickens. Chickens do not know how to and cannot fly."

Purpose

This book will disagree with just about everything you have learned, as is explained throughout this book. It is time to make changes in order to get different results.

As a preamble, I present my spiritual point of view:

"We are not merely human beings!
We are spiritual beings inhabiting human bodies.
The body was given to us for our spiritual evolution,
and it is our duty to care for it."

The goal of this book is to bring an understanding of the functions of the body, the purpose of these functions, the performance of the body, and also intimate knowledge of those elements that serve the physical development that otherwise cause damage.

All of this knowledge was acquired during the period when I experienced the cure of a Glioblastoma Multiforme Cancer Level 4 in the brain. Coupled with that were the experiences that, although they brought about pain, also strengthened my resolve through the suffering. While still experiencing joy during the illness, I was able to work toward obtaining a cure.

The people who were cured, like me, were radical in applying my therapy. They approached the disease like an enemy by first changing the way they think. All of the cells in our body work according to the frequency of our thoughts.

To better understand the results that I obtained, along with others who followed the same regimen I had developed, I will let you know that I have since augmented other factors that I have discovered since the time I was cured.

We are all part of a divine mind,
a unique and universal mind from which
all understanding and knowledge that is or
ever will be is within our grasp.
The successful are those who connect with
this universal mind ...

Change In Metabolism

The earth is not simply a rock in space. It is a living cell. Because of this, it exists in the same capacity as the human body, "that of healing itself." But for that to happen, it is necessary to change our own metabolism and create our own alternatives. The earth brings about its own phenomena, such as "El niño," then "EL niña," and the last one, in the Atlantic, "El Pato." These phenomena are part of a change in the terrestrial metabolism of the earth. Researchers are unable to explain the various phenomena that have been quickly coming on the earth.

Like the Schumann resonance, the earth is undergoing transitions, just as our bodies must adapt to changes. Schumann resonance is the earth's heartbeat at a natural and constant frequency pulsing at 7.83 Hz. An interesting detail is that those same discoveries made in 1952 are quite different from those of June 2014, when the Russian observatory exhibited a sudden increase, with an average peak of 8.5 Hz, but reaching as high as 16.5 Hz on certain days. The researchers believe that humans who have been in a latent state for thousands of years will be waking up to a new era of mental evolution. Nowadays we see an extraordinary development in children that was not present in the past, but damage can ensue in this evolution when overwhelming emotions are increased in moments of passion or mental stress.

The earth is trying to adjust to the new frequencies vibrated by us, and today, we have the feeling that time is passing faster than normal. I read in an article by Manoela Z. Bruskatto, dated April 30, 2017, about the Schumann resonance that "time is not the only notion we have of acceleration." We now have access to free information via the internet, one of our most important assets, and because of that, there has been a huge increase in global awareness. We human beings are becoming increasingly spiritual and mentally more aware than ever before. Considering that everything that physically lives will die one day, and the earth is a living cell, it may be in its period of maturation, or old age, like any other living thing because it is a living cell, and one day it too will die … without a doubt. We will not see this in our day, but this physical transformation does exist, and we hope it will occur in the very distant future. But this moment is a period of evolution, of transformation in everything and everyone who lives here. We may live a little longer than we did in years past, but only those who have the source of life in perfect condition will be able to enjoy the benefit of having a longer life.

The source of life is the blood because blood is life, and life is in blood. It is the blood that makes atonement for life (Leviticus 17:11). In this way, I dedicate myself more and more to helping people to clean their blood. The analysis of live blood is of supreme importance so that we can discover the things that can ruin the flesh. If the blood is dirty, the flesh rots, and diseases are the rot in the body. If the blood is clean, no disease remains in the body. Children who were born about three years ago are not prone to acquire the same diseases adults were prone to contract due to the change in metabolism. They were born with the new metabolism of the earth. We older ones, unfortunately, do not have this new metabolism! We need to adapt, and cleaning the blood makes it happen more quickly.

Take, for example, some executives who travel from the West to the East, and when they get there, they get sick. They immediately think that it was some food that hurt them. However, the body did not have time to adapt. Conversely, certain Orientals who come to the West also get sick soon after they arrive. We see the same situation here, as they did not have immediate adaptation. When we travel to extremely high or low places, our bodies need to adapt, or we will feel dizzy. I went through this problem many years ago in La Paz. I went down the stairs of the plane very fast and was hit with incredible dizziness. However, I got better right after having a glass of water and resting.

It seems like a joke, but let's analyze our body using the similarity of the terrestrial globe: When we have an illness or a simple virus, what does the body do? It creates fever. Fever is not a disease but a consequence and a warning system. If the earth is heating up, what do you think the viruses of the earth are? We are! Then we will see that our bodies were created with the three basic capacities: Cleaning itself … to heal itself … to adapt. That's what I mean.

Since I mentioned children, it is good to remember that no matter how adult we are, we have a child within us who needs to be well so that our adult well-being remains in balance.

There are times when the child asks for affection, needs an ice cream, needs to shout, spill, smile, or cry. We often need to attend to it, and never forget that it needs to be polite. If we allow it to have everything it wants, the results are sure to be catastrophic for the body.

Nothing in excess!

Everything in life has its parameters of balance.

- No excess food because you can get fat.

- No excess drink because it will generate addiction.

- No excess rest because it will create laziness.

- No excess exercise because it will wear out your body.

- No excess work because it will generate exhaustion.

- No excess anger that will turn to hate.

- No excess sadness because it will generate depression.

The only excess that is allowed is LOVE!

Our body was not created
with the intention that we must take vitamins;
our body is responsible for producing them for itself.
In order for that to happen,
we need to give it the raw materials
that produce them through digestion.

The Body Has Rules

*T*he most practical way I have found to explain that the body dictates the rules is as follows: Take a blender and put in some fruit juice, coconut water, or even some type of milk or pure water. Add a little cabbage, acerola, spinach, apple, cucumber, etc. Beat and make it a green juice that for many is perfect, right? Now, let's see if this juice is really perfect.

Approximately 15 to 20 minutes after drinking it, you should burp. You will not burp everything that was in the juice, but only the taste of one of the ingredients. Let us use as an example "the cucumber." The body internally separated what it does not need or has no biological function or does not do you good, and sent the taste into your mouth through the burp, which is the information that it no longer wants that food. However, you do not understand and continue adding cucumber.

Then more messages are sent causing a slight stomach upset, but you do not understand and keep eating the cucumber. The body returns with another message and makes you feel slightly dizzy, but the use of cucumber continues. There is a small allergy, with some itchiness on the body. However, you still do not get the message and continue to eat the cucumber. A new message is sent, and you feel a slight disturbance in your eyes as your sight becomes blurry. But it passes quickly, and you continue to eat the cucumber. The body sends one more message: It creates a small cold sore in the mouth. You take a dose of bicarbonate, and you are fine. But you keep on eating the cucumber. One more message and heartburn is triggered. You take an antacid and get better but keep eating the cucumber. At that moment, the body sends another message and makes you feel a headache. You take an aspirin, and it gets better. In the meantime, you keep eating the cucumber! Exhausted from sending so many messages, the body starts to weaken and sends you one more messase. You feel tired and discouraged but still eat the cucumber.

There comes a time when the body gets tired for good and sends the last warning message: ***"Now I'm going to get sick, so you can take care of me. Ready?"***

Now you are sick and will see a doctor who will order laboratory tests to find out what you have as a disease and to be able to medicate you.

At this moment, the *death ceremony* begins. I take this opportunity to explain what the death ceremony looks like through what Doctor L. I wrote.

Death Ceremony

The *death ceremony* began a long time ago as a simple ritual. In recent years, it has been developed by science. It usually takes 10 to 15 years. However, modern scientific advances are shortening this period of time.

It all starts with a simple aspirin for a simple headache. When one aspirin is no longer effective for the headache, you start taking two. After a few months, two aspirins become ineffective, and you take a stronger medicine. Then it is necessary to take something for the ulcers that were caused by the aspirin.

Now that you are taking two medications, you have a good start. After a few months, these drugs will disrupt the most important function, that of the liver.

If a good infection develops, you can take penicillin. Of course, penicillin will damage your red blood cells and spleen, and that's when you develop anemia. Now another drug is taken to cure anemia.

Thereafter, all of these medications will create tension in your kidneys, which will begin to fail in their functions. It is now time to take some antibiotics.

I would like to take this opportunity to explain what the ceremony of death is otherwise through what Dr. L. I. wrote.

"When these antibiotics destroy your intestinal flora and natural resistance, you can expect a general worsening of your symptoms. The next step is to cover all of these symptoms with controlled sulfa drugs. When the kidneys are finally damaged, you can drain. Some poisons will appear in your system, but you can continue to live for a long time that way. Now the medications you have taken will get your system so confused that they don't know what they have damaged, and they won't know what they have to fight either. But it really doesn't matter. You have followed all the steps here, and you can now make an appointment with your Creator. This game is played by practically everyone, with the exception of some ignorant people who just … Follow Nature."

By Dr. L. I

When the cause of the disease is removed, the body is able to heal itself.

Most people create erroneous realities and erroneously live those realities thinking they are right.

What Comes From The Outside Is Danger

The human body has an incredible ability to survive. As an example, let's look at a boat:

In the past, a boat was built only of wood because wood floats, and consequently, the boat would float. Today, however, we build ships and boats with iron and steel, but it does not sink with all the water around it. What makes the boat sink is the water that enters it.

What comes from the outside to the inside of the body is what will cause the damage if the body is not expelling or throwing out.

When we were children (of course, I am talking to people from the age of mercurochrome), if we had a cut or any skin injury, our mothers would coat it with mercurochrome, or "chrome mercury," and the wounds would heal very quickly. In one of my seminars in a hospital, I asked the doctors present why it was that when we put the mercury on the skin, the wounds would heal. I had several scientific pharmaceutical conflicting responses to the question. For example: mercury had a substance that healed wounds. But I was not told that mercury was harmful to the body. The body always maintains a little mercury that we acquire through food and/or environmental exposure.

You just can't retain it in excess.

So, I presented my knowledge of what I discovered about mercury. Although it healed wounds, the pharmaceutical industry no longer allowed chromium mercury sales in pharmacies because it was harmful to the body. When the chromium mercury was placed on wounds, the body reacted immediately, sending defenses so that the mercury would not penetrate. The wounds would heal very quickly because the white blood cells attacked the mercury, creating a barrier, and healing the wounded area so that other germs, or harmful bacteria or parasites, did not penetrate through the wound. We left the era of mercury, which did not burn when it was placed on wounds, to the era of Merthiolate, which burned painfully and took time to heal.

As evil comes from outside, let us look at the mind and the body in a similar way. Some of you may have watched vampire films. The vampire enters a house only if the owner invites him. He is evil, and evil cannot enter. We allow it to penetrate through the thoughts, creating emotions that are out of control, and causing us to make decisions that are completely harmful to us and to those without. Evil enters, begins to cause damage, and makes us mentally blind. I call that mental blindness. But this blindness can be cured, just by wanting to change. In fact, there is a phrase in English that I love:

"It's time to change."
Which means: It's time to change!

Allowing The Entry Of Evil

This is Humanity's Biggest Mistake!

*A*llowing it to happen ... we always allow it.

Everyone needs your permission: the mechanic who is going to fix your car, the plumber who is going to fix your sink, the doctor who is going to examine you, the waiter who is going to serve you, and the housekeeper who is going to clean your house. Lastly, everything you need you allow, everything!

All people voluntarily allow the body to get sick. Really, they do. Evil only comes in if you allow it. Diseases begin with things that enter the body, mainly harmful foods that have no biological benefit and can cause damage. Or, diseases begin with foods that are not harmful but that do not properly digest and, therefore, *become* harmful. Even allowing foreign bodies to enter ... our body aims to fight them immediately using our defense system, eliminating them through the dispatching organs.

During these years of taking care of many sick people, I always do a questionnaire before starting the blood analysis. With this, I have noticed that most of them had emotional problems caused by different reasons. The main one that affected their emotional state was the lack of love. It could be a lack of love for themselves or for other people. It could be because they felt rejected, or they expressed rejection for others. Some were people who did not like their bodies or the places where they lived. Some were not satisfied with their jobs or with their companions. Most usually always had a reason to be unhappy, even without knowing or remembering the reasons. Sorrow, as well as hatred and self-pity, have always been the reasons for a lack of love, and the body has always been the one to receive the negative results created by those emotions.

They are people who complain about the attitudes of others, who complain about the lack of attention, of the government's policies, work, the boss, fear of becoming poor, fear of losing something, etc.

The most interesting thing is that all these reasons lead to only one place:

The Lack of Love

It is important to remember that all the cells in our body work according to the vibrations created by our thoughts. An annoyance at the time of a meal can cause a stroke or a heart attack, but constant negative thinking is sure to cause the body to deteriorate.

Digestion
Verses
Bad Digestion

When digestion does not occur normally, the body has stopped metabolizing food properly. When the metabolism is functioning normally, the body produces and retains salts, vitamins, metals, and everything else it needs that is necessary to stay alive.

If we continue to maintain digestive deficiency, it will certainly not happen, and life will be shortened.

From now on, we must be concerned with maintaining a healthy body.

We don't have to worry about the body's past. The past has passed!

**WE NEED TO PREPARE A BETTER BODY
FOR THE FUTURE.**

Body Capacities

*O*ur body was created with three basic capacities: The first is to be able to *clean* itself. The second is to *heal* itself in order to *adapt*, which is the third capacity.

A healthy body is the body's ability to adapt to any circumstance. Our body has a similarity to the cockroach that adapts even to atomic radiation.

CLEAN • HEAL • ADAPT

Everything Is Three

Everything about strength comes from the number three (3). If we pay attention to engineering in buildings, we have the triangular system representing the force = 3.

Although the pyramids have four walls, each is formed by a triangle = 3. Our body has three capacities: **cleaning** itself, **healing** itself, and **adapting** = 3.

Darwin, "the notable" of evolutionists, said: "They will survive, not the strongest nor the most intelligent … They will survive, the most adaptable …"

There are three basic foods for humans: protein, fat, and **sugar** = 3. *(See later when I talk about food—what sugar, protein, and fat refer to. It will be what causes the bad digestion on page 101.)*

We have three basic sending organs = 3.
The **Colon** (bad things are expelled through the feces), the **Kidneys** (bad things come out through the urine), and the **Lungs** (bad things come out through the breath).

Of course, this is not to mention other dispatching bodies, such as the eyes that serve not only to see, but also to dispatch tears. I searched the Google library for something about the tears and found that there is only information concerning the physical part of the body. They forgot to add the emotional part with more clarification. The most I found simply informs that sadness causes tears. The tears that undoubtedly serve to clean the inside of the eyes and the parts of the lids that remain inside, are also to expel the feelings of sadness that can occur when our emotions are extremely affected. In reality, tears are not only caused by feelings of sadness, but also joy because we often cry with joy, which justifies that it is not only sadness that causes the tears, but that emotions are responsible for creating tears. The emotional works as a preventative by creating a forward defense so that foreign bodies do not enter the visual field, even when some speck or burning gets into the eyes. That is the glory of being able to see.

The tear is also the dispatch of a very harmful acid to the body, so it needs to leave. People who are unable to cry are usually emotionally tough, and their metabolism is unable to create tears. Don't be ashamed to cry.

ARE YOU TOO SHY TO CRY? ... CRY!

This is good for your body, so that the harmful acids can come out and not create moments of anger, rancor, or extreme sadness. Feelings can make the body sick and vulnerable because all of the cells in our body work according to vibrations created by our thoughts. The Indians have a very interesting way of not allowing sadness to occupy a long space in their minds. If they lose a loved one, they cry for three straight days. They are then ready to go on with life without the presence of the loved one.

Many people prefer to remain in suffering. They forget that life goes on. I have had some losses in my life. First, it was my father, then my mother, and finally, my wife. I cried those losses, but, as we cannot go back to the past to start all over again, I decided to create another future.

> *We don't have to worry about the past.*
> *The past has passed!*
> *We need to prepare for a better future.*
> (Chico Xavier)

Longing
Is The Love That Stays

We need to remember that nostalgia is the love that remains, or love is the nostalgia that remains, and that is yours. It is you. It is the symbol of a beautiful feeling.

We can regret the loss, but we cannot stop in the space of suffering. The best mental capacity that God gave to human beings was to be able to love again, always again. We will be loving other people, other jobs, other goals, other achievements, always with different intensity.

These are trials that are given to us for our spiritual evolution. To perpetuate suffering is to deteriorate the mind. This will deteriorate the body, leading to physical succumbing and mental weakness, which can lead to suicide.

At this point, it is good to remember that *the only sin that cannot be forgiven is suicide*. The person will be struggling against the life of someone who has no defense: the self!

If there is such a loss in your life, cry for three days. Remember that love is the longing that remains. That feeling is the purest and most sublime of all the feelings that you can have.

When we cry, we calm down. Feelings of losing love can

be cried, but not for too long. Even the trees cry after pruning, but they react with new growth. God gave the human being the incredible ability to always be able to love again.

Let's go back to talking about number three:

- "You are valiant, brave, and fearless" = 3.
  So, be a human being: Cry!
- We have *physical receptors:* sight, smell, and touch = 3.
- As *basic factors, the elements:* earth, air, and water = 3.
- As *consequential elements:* heat, cold, and comfort = 3.
- As *energetic elements:* hate, love, and fear = 3.
- As *physical elements:* the body, trunk, and limbs = 3.
- *Subdividing the body:* arm, forearm, and hand = 3.
- *In the hand:* carpus bones, metacarpal bones, and phalanges (fingers) = 3.
- *In the fingers:* proximal, medial, and distal phalanx = 3.
- *As origin:* the beginning, the middle, and the end = 3.
- *Movements:* forward/back, side to side, up/down = 3.

Let's look at this aspect of the three groups of life:

- Waking, living, and resting = 3.
- Ingesting, digesting, and extracting = 3.
- Sleeping, working, and having fun = 3.
- Dreaming, imagining, and executing = 3.

We have 24 hours in a day divided into three periods:

• Eight hours to rest, eight hours to work, eight hours to have fun = 3.

Not everyone can stay in these numbers because, in reality, almost nobody obeys these details of life. Some work too much. Others don't work at all. Others rest too much. And few really have fun in the one-third period reserved for fun because, for the most part, they are stressed, disturbed, unhappy with life, suffering, and many are cholerically disturbed. They forget that everything in life, including happiness, is a matter of decision. They do not remember that the only decision that cannot be made is not to make a decision. "Be happy."

Roman Emperor Marcus Aurélius spoke a phrase that few remember and most are unaware of: *"We become what we think and speak."*

And if we look a little more spiritually, we have: THE FATHER, SON, and HOLY SPIRIT. Is it a coincidence, or does it say something? Your future is determined by who you honor. The world is in the hands of those who have the ability to dream and take the risk of living out their dreams.

Body Sending Bodies

In order for the body to perform its own healing, it must first:

Cleanse itself
Heal itself
Be able to adapt

The cleaning processes are developed through:
- THE COLON - Eliminating impurities through feces.
- THE KIDNEYS - Eliminating impurities by urine.
- THE LUNGS - Eliminating impurities via breathing.
- THE SKIN is the largest extracting organ, where allergies are reflected in the skin. Spots, itches, and wounds that appear in the skin are part of the lymphatic system expelling and identifying impurities, toxins that cannot stay inside us, warning that something is not right in the physiological system, or bacteria or viruses or toxins that the defenses are not destroying, or some food without biological function was introduced through food or even through breathing.

It is necessary to understand a little more about cures because people misinterpret medications. For example, if you have an infection, you go to the doctor. He prescribes an antibiotic. You go to the pharmacy, buy the antibiotic, go home, take it, get the improvement, and attribute it to the medicine. But the antibiotic does not cure anyone. It stops the growth of the germ, bacteria, virus, parasite, etc. The defense, which is the white blood cells, is what comes to the cure because if we do not have the white blood cells, which are the body's defense, there will be no healing associated with the lymphatic system that will work on the expedition.

Let's look at the case of people who get sick with AIDS. They do not die of AIDS. They die from a simple cold because they no longer have white blood cells as a defense. I would also like to emphasize a detail about AIDS that I discovered in recent years.

HIV is an acronym in English for Human Immuno-deficiency Virus, a virus that causes a deficient or weakened immune system. HIV can be treated and is effective if the treatment is followed consistently. It is known that if HIV is not treated, it can progress to AIDS, Acquired ImmunoDeficiency Syndrome. The virus spreads everywhere in the body, but AIDS goes to one organ only. AIDS chooses the white blood cells, the main line of the body's defense system. AIDS has the characteristic of a parasite more than a virus because parasites reside in and kill defense cells. If the human system is corrupted and weak with little defense or without the ability to proliferate more defense, each white cell that it attacks means one less cell to perform the necessary defense work for the body.

People often say that such and such a person died of AIDS. What really happened is that the person infected with HIV that became large scale in the body did not die of AIDS. They died, perhaps, of a simple cold. The virus called HIV, already in large scale in the body, enabled AIDS to overtake the cells in the defense system, killing the white blood cells. We cannot survive without this defense.

Returning to the purpose of this information, the person may have HIV in the body, but if the body is healthy with the capacity to always create the necessary number of defenses, it will never be sick. But for this to happen, it will be necessary for the entire system to be properly powered.

Digestion Is Everything

The body will be fed if all food ingested has also been properly digested. If the organic system is able to use digested food to supply the physiological needs of the body, everything will be fine. The big problem is that when something does not digest, it stays and accumulates. If we digest, everything that follows from there will be beneficial to the body.

As an example, let us look at two dominoes. The white row represents good digestion.

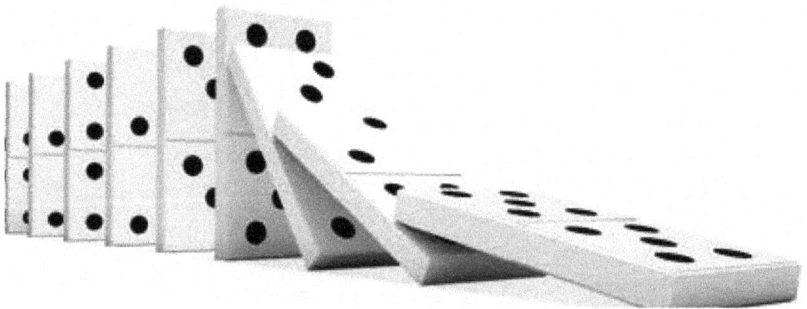

But if the first stone of another color that represents a bad digestion is pushed, all other actions of the body will follow the same path (bad things generate other bad things).

There begins the process of malnutrition. In this case, it is the mutations that cause transformations to cease to exist.

**The other color row
represents poor digestion.
The taste of victory is only known
when we discover that we have tried.**

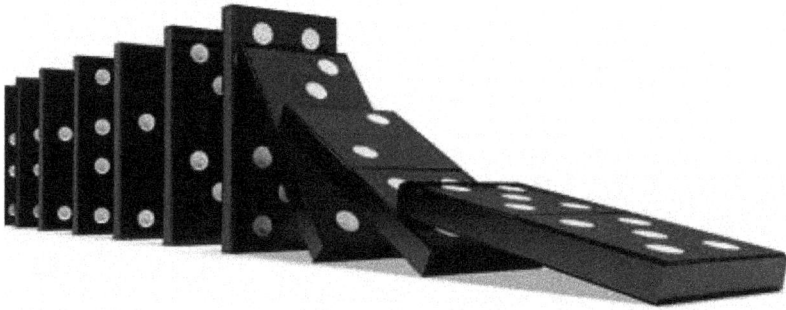

According to Lavoisier's theory, "On the face of the earth, nothing is lost, nothing is created, everything is transformed." And, we need to understand that our body was created for transformations. However, due to the unfavorable internal environment, these transformations will cease to exist, creating the mutations, which will cause illness.

In the book *"BÉCHAMP OR PASTEUR?"* subtitled *"Pasteur: Plagiarist, impostor"* by Ethel Douglas Hume, with the Germ theory that was in evidence to benefit the Pharmaceutical Industry, he puts a lot of information in his book, important info that the world does not know because it decided to believe in the Pharmaceutical Industry and in the works of Louis Pasteur, when Béchamp's work was the most important.[1] In the book above, he explains where and how Pasteur, who was a disciple of Béchamp, mistakenly changed the fate of the world when he brought to the pharmaceutical industry the experience of what is otherwise known by Béchamp, of the germ fighting germ, creating the so-called "antibiotic," which means "anti-life."

---

1 **Review Note:**
The germ theory of Pasteur and his contemporaries.

In 1800, I saw three prominent scientists who were involved, in different ways, of the same topic. One of his books is *Dr. Pasteur* (1822-1895), noted for his germ theory steeped in mainstream theory. Unlike his contemporaries, Pasteur was rich in making his theory predominant, as he knew the Jewish person and was very influential he himself. According to this theory, we do not come in contact with infected microorganisms from outside our body. A specific species of microbe can attack the body of the sternum and cause a specific disease. Today, the medical profession is based on this theory and operates of succeeds: for a specific microbe a specific medicinal cure is preceded. The monomorphism is that theory that maintains that the microorganism does not change in any case the form or the species. Pasteur is also noted for not having been trapped in any consideration, in his theory of germs, the scope of his contemporary colleges. One of them. the second scientist in question, is Dr. Claude Bernard (1813-1878), whom generally no one today has ever heard of. His scientific studies show how the most important factor in the matter was the internal environment, which is important for the first time described as the internal environment. The body gets sick only when the internal "ground" has lost its balance or homeostasis. Scientific third dealing with this subject of Antoine Béchamp (1816-1908), the theory starts from this foundation of Bernard. Also according to Béchamp, the disease occurs when our internal ground is unbalanced. He showed, moreover, that a non-equilibrium internal ground causes a pleomorphic reason. The microbiologicals, already present in the form of microzymes, are observed by the scientist as they transform into bacteria, mold or fungi and vice versa (polymorphism), depending on their environment.

Check if this process is necessary, it is necessary that the circostant is an acidic environment. The polymorphism was successively studied and proven by many other scholars. One of these, for example, Dr. Rife, has not studied the impact of cancer. Many of his claims were silenced and all his writings and laboratory equipment were destroyed, in 1939. Gaston Naesson is another scientist who has explored and publicized the pleomorphic activity and the flu that this has the environment in which it is found.

If the germ theory were founded, why isn't every color that comes into contact with the microbomb that forms? An immediate example is that a graduate student in a class of three students. They will never all get sick. We need to explore the question further. Why? One answer might be that the unloved student has a stronger immune system.

Another, like the first, states that the surrounding environment did not allow the microbes to form. Taken from: http://www.seniorchiropratica.it/pasteur-e-i-suoi-contemporanei/.

That is, life destroying life, not allowing the origin of creation, which is the transformations, to do its normal healing work. Béchamp, in his discoveries made with germs, made it very clear that since the body has the ability to heal itself, it should always be healthy, and for that it would be necessary to take care of the body, always keeping it with the ability to defend itself only, and it would not be necessary to create different foreign bodies in the body, which could cause damage to other organs not affected by possible infections. Pasteur, a disciple of Béchamp, used this knowledge of Béchamp to publicize the experiences made with Germs and that is how the greatest beneficiary of this knowledge became richer and more powerful: "The pharmaceutical industry."

So, today, due to people's preference for using the resources of the pharmaceutical industry, they forget that the body has the ability to heal itself. Obviously, after we deteriorate our defenses, our body is at the mercy of the enemy that proliferates day after day with mutations that will originate more diseases in organs that would never be damaged if we had understood and took care of our bodies, and obeyed their messages. If we did, none of this would happen.

**Nothing is lost, nothing is created,
everything is transformed.
Nothing is a reason for death.
Everything is the reason for life.**
By Antoine Béchamp

Body Transformations

For the above to be understood, it is interesting to note that we are as microorganisms that turn into bacteria, that turn into fungi, that turn, that turn, that turn … until the body has no need to transform. The lymphatic system will be expelling what no longer serves, or the excess, through the sending organs.

The skin, being also an excretory organ, serves to show that there is an excess, or something that the body has not digested, and/or was unable to expel through the three main organs. Another possibiity is that it has no biological function in the body and needs to be expelled because it has undergone mutations and did not follow the normal transformation process.

At this moment, there are several diseases that can appear, such as: melasma; white cloth; seborrheic dermatitis; rosacea; alopecia areata; dyshidrosis; folliculitis; allergy; fungi ringworm of the skin, foot, and nail; atopic dermatitis; psoriasis; scabies; as well as skin cancer and many others. Our influences are created and transmitted to others, so we need to ensure they are positive.

The External Wound
Is An Expedition

I saw a patient, Vilma dos Santos Sá, who had wounds on her legs for a long time and was unable to get a cure. During the blood analysis, I found a number of fungi that had mutated with fermentation and infection, as well as toxins from the feces, and I explained that the wound was the body itself trying to expel the impurities. She was radical, strictly complied with my therapeutic suggestions, and in a short time, her wounds disappeared completely. See below the pictures of her legs before and after the blood had been cleaned.

With Wounds

Only Scars

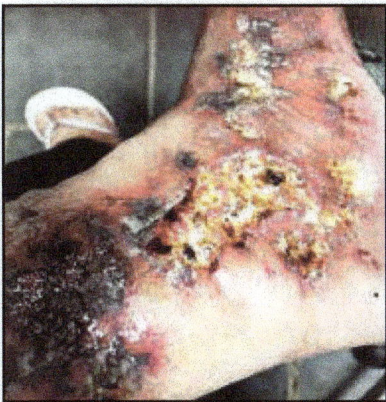 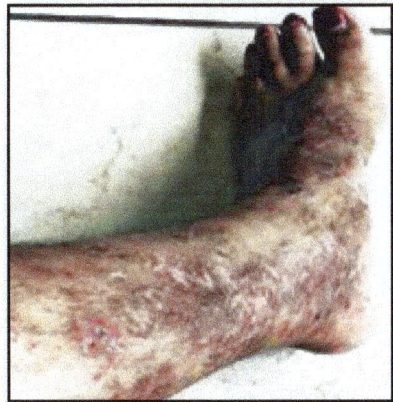

Following is the lovely letter from Vilma dos Santos Sá:

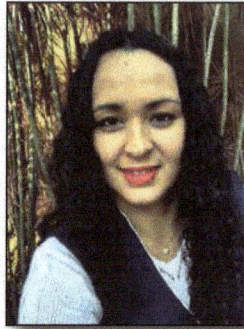

Vilma dos Santos Sá

Dear Dr. Jimmy,
Allow me to call you a Doctor because you are a
doctor at what you do. I give you permission to add
this to your book, and would really like my testimony
and thanks to be part of your book so that people who
may be experiencing health problems, as I did, know
that Dr. Jimmy Albuquerque with his therapy works
miracles. For years with medical treatments I never
obtained the healing results, but today, after I met
with him, and had the treatment with his therapy, I
am very happy because now I am able to carry out
activities such as work and sport, leisure, all without
limitations. The time of suffering is over. My feet and
legs really healed. The only thing that bothers a little
are the scars, but in view of what I have been through
for years, this is the least. I will never forget what
you did for me. Today I am sure that my health
problems are gone. I am a healthy woman. I thank
God for putting you, Dr. Jimmy, in my life.
Vilma dos Santos Sá
Sao Paulo 09/13/2019

A Light Scientific Explanation

Many people have chronic wounds and complain, but in reality, they should thank God that they are there on the skin, outside, because if the wound is inside the body, the problem is much more serious. If the body is unable to clean itself completely, the excess impurities that accumulate will make normal healing processing difficult because the defense organs, such as the white blood cells and the lymphatic system that have the function of protecting, will be occupied with other tasks, uncovering the areas that need constant maintenance. Neutrophils, which are able to leave blood vessels and penetrate tissues attacking bacteria and other foreign bodies, as well as Eosinophils that proliferate when allergic reactions occur, or there is an increase in parasites in the body, and Basophils that also work on allergic responses, including dilating and permeabilizing blood vessels and monocytes, which are white cells that become macrophages (large), which also enter tissues to ingest other substances foreign to the body that are possibly harmful to the body. In order to understand a little more about white cells (leukocytes), the deficiency can cause damage by attacks of parasites, harmful bacteria to our body, while the excesses show that there is already some infection or inflammation in the body. Neutrophil is a type of white blood cell, that is, white cells that work as defenses fighting mutations, usually caused by the lack of oxygen in the affected areas. When we find excesses of white blood cells in the analysis of live blood, we can conjecture some physical divergence such as recent surgeries and uses of certain drugs.

Definitely the excesses found in the analysis of living blood shows that there is already something to be fought such as infections caused by bacteria or fungi in a mutated state. There are some stages in fungi when the body's internal environment is not favorable (lack of oxygen). In fungal fermentation, the candida is created, and in the second stage of the mutation comes the fungal infection. In the analysis of the live blood, we see that it expands with a nucleus and tentacles that do not allow the red blood cells (RBC)[2] to reach them. In that case, only white blood cells can attack them. At this point, it is worth remembering that red blood cells carry oxygen, and the only thing that lives without oxygen in acidic environments in our body is cancer.

(This information and the technical terms are necessary here, so that you can understand the body's defenses.)

Knowledge only has value when the mind is prepared.

---

2 **Review Note:**
 Red blood cells (RBCs), also known as erythrocytes, are circulating blood cells responsible for transporting oxygen throughout the body. The RBC count quantifies the total number of red blood cells in an individual's blood. It is one of the parameters included in the CBC examination and is often used in assessing a person's general health status.

The defenses, (white blood cells) should be protecting the body from other harmful bodies such as viruses, parasites, germs, mutant bacteria, but because of unfavorable internal environments created by poor digestion, the white cells are completely busy working on the undigested food residues. They should always be available to deal with the dangers, which are parasites, germs, viruses, and mutated bacteria. The white blood cells will spend much more time working on the poor digestion of food, when they should dedicate themselves to the destruction of the harmful elements that our body will be vulnerable to acquire.

Our bodies and all our cells work according to the vibrations created by our thoughts.

What Is Digestion

In order to understand this moment, we need to understand what digestion is: stomach acids are responsible for digesting food that will become feces, releasing food for a second stage of digestion. Most oral acids are responsible for the digestion of food. There are thousands of foods, but only three foods for our bodies.

PROTEIN – used for the growth of new cells. For example, the soles of our feet as well as the palms of our hands will never wear out, because that is how we were created for producing new cells. It is worth mentioning that many people try to ingest protein from industrialized products, and this is a mistake because, at first, our body was not created to take chemicals nor vitamins. It has the ability to create these necessary cells, vitamins, and nutrients as long as we have a good digestion of the foods and the nutrition that is in the foods.

FAT – which is also in foods, and serves for general lubrication of our body, serves to lubricate the veins, our joints, our eyes, our mouth, and our entire flexible system. Anyway, if there was no fat in the body, we would be rigid.

(This was the simplest way I found to explain the need for "fat" food). Take, for example, the case of poor digestion of fats, which create plaques that lodge inside arteries, clogging arteries that can cause stroke. And once it is not digested, it will stop lubricating the artery walls. When the heart pulls blood through the artery to send it to the lungs, the blood moves with speed, causing uric acid and or cholesterol, which are sharp crystals, to scratch the vein walls, creating coronary infection.

SUGAR – Before explaining the importance of sugar, I want to clarify that all food also contains sugar, which is itself a type of food, in addition to fat and protein. Everything that comes out of the earth (understood as the terrestrial globe), has the three necessary foods to be alive: Protein, Fat and Sugar = 3. We don't need any other industrialized sugar. What is in the natural foods do not hurt, even for those who have cancer. I know this because when I was sick, I ate a lot of fruit in its natural state. Important note: Those who have cancer cannot eat any dried or cooked fruit, because when the fruit is dried or cooked, it separates the sugar from the fructose. The person will be ingesting the sugar separately from the fructose, which in this case is food for cancer. Sugar acidifies the body, and it is also good to remember that cancer can live in extremely acidic environments.

In passing, the most addictive drug for humans is sugar, then heroin, and then cocaine. The sugar ingested through natural foods will be transformed into calcium for the bones and energy for the body. If the body is digesting these three foods, it will not be necessary to use vitamins sold in pharmacies, created by laboratories. I emphasize that God created our body with the three basic capacities: Cleaning itself to heal itself, and being able to adapt. Our body was not created to take vitamins. It, the body, has the capacity to produce the vitamins, salts, and substances necessary for its perfect performance, if we give it the raw material for this production, which is the digestion of the three foods: protein, fat, and sugar. Poor digestion was and is the cause of illness.

Hence, the title and subtitle of this book:

We are *not* what we eat.
We *are* what we do not digest and assimilate.

Basic Organs

The evolution of the times and the need for economic development have led us to start industry, which has been changing and devolving our lives, creating many industrialized foods that are harmful to our bodies. We can live without many of our organs and limbs, such as the spleen, gallbladder, appendix, prostate, uterus, ovaries, tubes, penis, arms, and legs. We can live like human trunks without all of these organs, but we cannot live without the major organs that fail to perform their functions, such as the liver, pancreas, lungs, and kidneys. Death, which is cardiac arrest, has its origin in diseases in different major organs.

The heart, a simple pump, can also be damaged by the consequences of undigested food. It is the only one that never has cancer because it is in constant activity. What normally damages the heart is an excess of uric acid crystals and/or bad cholesterol (which are sharp crystals that are in excess in the blood).

Remember that, in life, everything
is a matter of balance, and nothing
in excess is good for our body.

When the heart pulls blood into it, the blood comes with speed, and if the fat has not been properly digested, it will stop lubricating the inside walls of the arteries. These sharp crystals scratch the walls of the heart's internal arteries, creating coronary infections. Again, poor digestion is present as causing premature death. As I explained earlier, there are thousands of foods available to our body, but only three (3) basic foods: Protein, Fat, and Sugar.

Remember that when I talk about Protein, Fat, and Sugar, I am not referring to industrialized products but to what was given to us as food by the Creator.

Everything that exists on earth for our body's survival has these three basic foods:

Protein, Fat, and Sugar

For example: if you do not have food at home, you can eat grass. Contrary to popular opinion, you won't die, because grass has protein, fat, and sugar. (Let it register that the cow only eats grass and still gets fat!) Stomach acids are responsible for digesting the food that will release the food that was in the food and will be directed to feed the liver and pancreas, which are the two main organs for metabolizing food.

The digestion of food produces nutrition. It will be sent to the liver and pancreas, which will do their job of metabolizing so the body is fed. The last result in the digestion of food will be feces, debris that no longer interests the body.

Enzymes are essential for every function of the human body that produces over 3,000 of its own enzymes. These facilitate work connected to the nervous system, functions of the digestive system, functions of the immune system, blood cells, lactation, reproduction, and transformations.

All foods when raw contain the enzymes necessary to break them down and pre-digest them before the body does. When digestion is not achieved by a normal process through the enzymes contained in the raw food itself, the body needs to bring its enzymes to do its job and finish the digestion process. When food is heated above 118 ° or subjected to low temperatures, salts and heavy metals, as well as ultraviolet radiation or dehydration, destroy natural enzymes. More demand is then deposited on the body to put its own enzymes in greater quantities to continue the digestion process and uncovers several areas making them vulnerable to disease. It is ideal to ingest a high percentage of enzymes in our diet, but for most people this is impractical considering their busy lifestyles.

So, what is the answer, the solution to that? It is natural `enzymes, such as malt diastasis, Amyloglucosidase, Invertase, Lipase, Neutral protease, Fungal protease, Acid Stable protease, Cellulase, Hemicellulose, Fungal Lactase and Fungal Amylase. These are found in some food supplements produced by some laboratories. The best enzyme food supplement I used when I was cured had all of the enzymes I would like to highlight here … the Enzimax produced in the United States, as well as other probiotics. Some raw foods contain enough enzymes to help digest, but there are other foods not produced by laboratories that serve to speed up digestion, such as papaya or pineapple, that can also help digest proteins as Bromolin does. We can eat papaya and pineapple at each meal, although it is not very practical.

One answer is Aspergillus[3] enzymes: broad-spectrum Aspergillus enzymes located in a wide range of pH 2-11 that work throughout the digestive tract. But if we drink liquids before meals, as some doctors and therapists say, these enzymes will no longer be available to complete digestion because they will be washed out and taken to the dispatching organs. Animals, for example, never drink before meals, nor during, nor after. They wait for digestion to happen. If drinking liquids before meals, it will be necessary to use enzymes found in food supplements, such as the ones I listed above.

---

3 **Review Note:** The main characteristics of **enzymes obtained from Aspergyllus** fungus can be summarized as follows:

They are active at a temperature approaching that of the human body, They can function in an environment ranging from Ph 3.0 to Ph 9.0 and are therefore the only enzymes active in both the acidic, basic and neutral tracts of the intestine. In this regard, it is important to note that Pepsin and Trypsin function only in the acidic Ph of the stomach, while pancreatic enzymes are active only in the alkaline Ph of the small intestine. Their activity already begins in the upper part of the stomach. This promotes a decrease in the body's own digestive enzyme secretion, allowing the pancreas to produce greater amounts of systemic and immune enzymes. In fact, food enzymes are "naturally" activated by heat already during chewing thus initiating the so-called "pre-digestion" process, which continues even as the food continues on its way to the stomach, only to be inactivated by gastric secretions. Later, the alkaline environment of the small intestine reactivates food enzymes that contribute to the completion of the digestive process. They effectively break down proteins, carbohydrates, fats, and fiber, unlike, for example, bromelain and papain, which have an exclusively proteolytic action. In addition, this special blend of digestive enzymes also allows them to break down sugars, dairy products, and even promote the assimilation of minerals contained in vegetables by the enzyme Endo-phytase.

Clarifying more popularly what is digestion, it is necessary to understand the elements necessary for the digestion of food (protein, fat, and sugar). The two places where there are more bacteria in our bodies are as follows: at the entrance to the mouth, and at the fecal extraction area, at the exit.

Oral bacteria, or enzymes that originate in the mouth, are used for the digestion of the foods that were in the food—protein, fat, and sugar. Consider this detail. If they are responsible for the digestion of food, then they must enter our body alive and not dead. Therefore, oral hygiene directed and ordered by the pharmaceutical industry is no longer necessary.

The Mouth Was Not Made To Be Washed

Animals do not wash their mouths because they know instinctively they need oral enzymes. You can brush your teeth after meals, but you don't need to wash or rinse your mouth. Brush with a dry or even wet brush and swallow. It's not crap! We bring worse things to our mouths! It does not! All oral enzymes, also called oral bacteria, were placed at the entrance that serve for the digestion of food. (I will explain later what is and what is not food.)

Sometimes people ask me if they can use dental floss. I usually make a joke and say: *Only on the beach!* Obviously, if something you chew gets caught between your teeth and is bothering you, take it out! Dear readers, divine creation is incredible. God did not create toothpaste. The pharmaceutical industry created it.

Have you discoveed a detail that has gone unnoticed by many people? There are now no *hard* toothbrushes in the world. The pharmaceutical industry has removed all *hard* toothbrushes from the market worldwide. You will find only *medium* and *soft*. In the United States, brush producers (pharmaceutical industry) were forced to launch beyond the *average* and the *soft* a brush that they labeled as *firm*. It is no longer the *hard fiber brush* (*harder* in English). It is now labeled as *FIRM*, deceiving the people! The explanation they give is that the medium and soft fiber brushes are used to massage the gums. But the ones that really clean are the most rigid and *hard* fiber brushes.

During a period of my life, I had the opportunity to live in other countries. When I lived in Nigeria, Africa, I had the opportunity to see many people with extremely white teeth. I saw that my driver had perfect, extremely white teeth. One day, I asked him if he brushed his teeth and what paste he used. He surprised me when he said he brushed, but he did not use toothpaste. I asked to see the brush he used and was even more surprised when I saw that it was a small stick, like an ice cream stick. He rubbed his teeth with this stick right after he ate. While I lived in Nigeria, I used this same type of wood as a brush without using toothpaste. I think it was great progress in my life because, after I stopped using toothpaste, I never had bad breath again. If God knew we would need to floss, He would have made a single plaque like teeth. If there is a gap between one tooth and another, it is for some reason. The food residues that remain will create other enzymes that, when ingested, will help digestion.

Everything that is at the entrance is to enter, everything that is at the exit is to leave.

Let us look at the not-so-remote past. In the past, there was no toothpaste. Animals do not brush their teeth. They don't have bad breath. They have breath, and that, we all have. If your digestion is not perfect, your breath will be sour and often give off the stink of undigested putrefied food, even if you put perfume in your mouth. But even if you have good digestion, the smell will come out a little bit sour. However, just drink a little water, and that will no longer smell the same.

Some people ask me if they should never brush their teeth. Please, my people! (Please, my people!) The large number of processed foods we eat, saturated fats, preservatives, chemicals, and sugars that now appear in these foods will certainly bring other substances that can adhere to the teeth and will have to be eliminated, as explained above. My suggestion is to brush your teeth before you go to sleep with coconut fat and baking soda, which is an abrasive to clean and brighten your teeth. At this time, if you want to wash your mouth, you can do so because, during the night, it will accumulate the enzymes necessary for the digestion of food that will be eaten the next day.

BAD BREATH IN THE MOUTH

Animals do not have cavities unless they are eating foods with sugar because what causes cavities is sugar. Take, for example, when domestic animals, such as the dog and the cat, ate the leftover food from the dining table.

Everyone died of old age. Today, they die of diseases, including cancer, because they are fed by industrialized rations that contain preservatives harmful to the animals' bodies, and ours as well.

> *The enzymes responsible for digestion are generally considered to be the light of life. They are necessary for all body functions. You ought to be asking the questions: Is this information worth considering? Does that say anything?*

Many serious health problems, such as arthritis, heart disease, gastrointestinal disorders, cancer, and other diseases, are caused because, every day, more and more people are forgetting to focus on preventing themselves from getting sick.

The body maintains a reserve of enzymes that cannot be less than necessary. If a person spends his enzymes quickly, he is sure to have a short life span! The most incredible thing is that the body does not have an immediate reaction to this problem created by the lack of enzymes. It gradually deteriorates and without pain. We do not pay attention until the deterioration is chronic and unable to be repaired.

At this point, the body becomes vulnerable to any disease. Poor digestion of food has priority for the body, which sheds its enzyme reserves for digestion, making many areas vulnerable without their natural defenses.

We usually only go to a doctor's office when we feel something is wrong. At this point, it is good to remember that once you have consulted the doctor, you will surely come out with a prescription to be dispatched and, consequently, will streamline the process of the death ceremony previously described in this book.

The good digestive functioning will make each nutrient absorbed by the organic system through the bloodstream, where organs, cells, and tissues will be constantly healthy, and in the process what no longer serves will be expelled. This is the basic process of creating our bodies: cleaning yourself. Perfect digestion is the fuel for the body's energetic and healthy life source. Poor digestion, on the other hand, if there is no perfect expedition work, will render areas of our body defenseless and will become a mutation within us and not transformation. Our body was created to have transformations and not mutations.

Digestion develops transformations.
Poor digestion causes mutations.

So, this process of mutation develops bacteria, making them harmful. They become toxic in our body; they spread and damage organs, cells, and tissues, initiating diseases and other illnesses. The intoxication caused by the mutations affects the organic functions creating weaknesses in the immune system, including making chronic fatigue, weakness, headaches, ulcers, allergies, and even the depression that is currently the evil that most plagues humanity.

During these ten years of work as a morphologist, I have come across many people who suffer from depression. When I analyze their blood in the microscope, I realize that, for the most part, they do not digest the food nor the protein of the foods they consume. In this sense, the red cells, the RBCs, do not carry the necessary amount of oxygen to the brain. This is not the only cause of depression, but it certainly contributes a lot.

About 20% of the oxygen that is acquired when the heart pumps blood to the lungs goes to the brain, and in this case, due to the erythrocytes not receiving oxygen in full because they are glued together, aggregated because of poor protein digestion, oxygen will be lacking, which is the source of life, in the brain, where problems can occur that can lead to a twisted mind.

Examples Of Good And Bad Blood

*L*et us look below at examples of good and damaged blood.

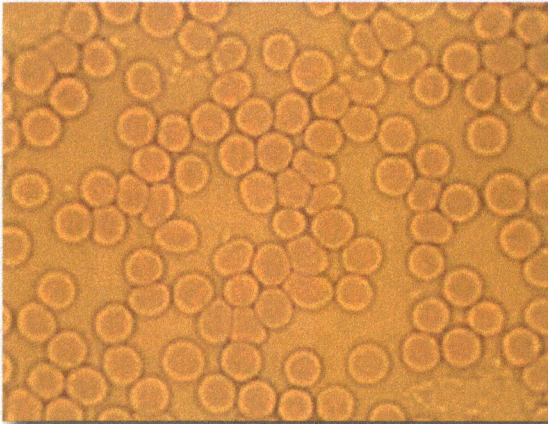

1-Good blood

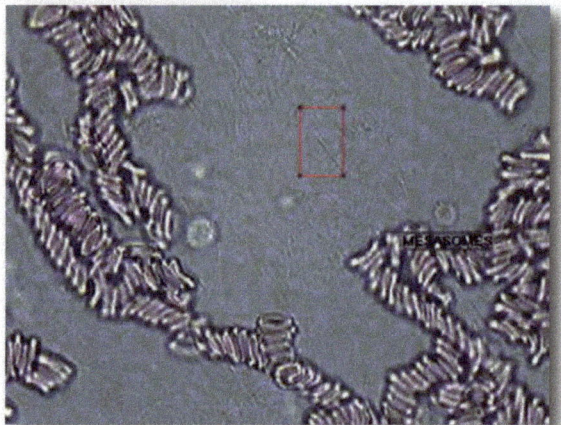

2-Bad blood

There are other types of irregularities in red blood cells. In cases like this, I suggest an immediate blood cleaning and a *coaching* treatment so that the blood cleaning is simultaneously changing with new incentives for a healthy mental and physical life, where the spiritual can accompany this evolution.

What you think, you create.
What you feel, you attract.
What you believe is true becomes fact.

The food industry directs us to eat foods through advertisements and multicolored commercials that are good at brainwashing, but they do not tell us that these foods, in addition to not containing toxin-free foods caused mostly by fertilizers or preservatives that are extremely harmful to our body, they can cause irreparable damage. Although some government agencies establish information requirements on packaging, they are in lower spectrum, and almost nobody cares to read this information, since they no longer appear in many products. People buy pasteurized food thinking it is good for their health, but they are not informed that food that has undergone a pasteurization process has been heated to extremely high temperatures, destroying any existing enzymes.

Once this type of food is ingested, the body has extra work for digestion using enzymes that should be looking for harmful elements. Instead, the enzymes that should be looking for harmful elements will now be used to aid digestion. People believe that pasteurizing food kills bacteria, but they do not understand what part of these bacteria are necessary for proper digestion to make the body healthy. In order for the body to remain healthy, digestion is required, and if food does not carry its own enzymes, it has to steal enzymes from the immune system, making some other part vulnerable to attacks by foreign elements that will definitely create damage that will cause disease. The lack of oxygen transmitted by red blood cells makes the body acidic, creating mutations. At this point, it is worth mentioning that the fungi are able to live in acidic environments that will undergo mutations giving rise, for example, to candida during the fermentation period of the fungi.

When the immune system becomes deficient, for various reasons caused by the lack of oxygen that originated from poor digestion, the red blood cells, now aggregated together, no longer carry the necessary amounts of oxygen in all parts of the body, weakening it. It now needs to use the defenses that went to work on digestion, making the system deficient. When digestion is not complete, the lack of oxygen will cause the transformations to cease to exist, giving rise to mutations. It has been more than proven that candidiasis that causes great discomfort in women, such as vaginal burning, discharge, itching, swelling, and possible fissures, are not sexually transmitted. It is a consequence of mutations that occur due to lack of oxygen and cause fungicidal mutations that spread on a large scale.

For women, because they are expelled through the vagina due to being in excess, they are not combated by the vaginal flora, causing discomfort in women who, in their majority, seek the most hygienic means possible to avoid and combat this discomfort. However, they forget that the vagina was not made to be washed with soap because it destroys the vaginal flora and can become chronic. Fungi and candida are the danger because they live in dark, humid, and hot environments. Do you want a better environment for them to develop and live in that is not inside our body, which is dark and damp? Fungi and candida feed on ingested and undigested sugar, which also causes Diabetes because the pancreas does not receive digested food and is deficient in its functions.

As for the heart, as I said before, it is not a food producing or metabolizing organ. It is a simple pump, and when we fill the lungs with oxygen, it sends blood to the lungs to receive oxygen and transport it throughout the body because oxygen is the source of life. However, if the fat, which is one of the three staples, does not digest properly, it stops doing the job of lubricating the artery walls. When the heart pulls the blood, it comes with speed, and the cholesterol and uric acid that are sharp crystals enter scratching the walls of the veins creating coronary infections. Now, the person will have heart problems! *(See on page 101 the Table of Diseases Caused By Poor Digestion.)*

It is worth talking a little about diabetes. Obviously, many people are already born with certain organ deficiencies

73

with a tendency to diseases such as diabetes, but most of the time, a simple blood test will show some sugar crystals, and that does not mean that the person is diabetic. The doctor says that he has a beginning of diabetes. Then he will prescribe medication, which will remove the function of the pancreas, and then, yes, diabetes will arise. The sugar crystals in the food go through a normal digestion process, but if the person ingested animal milk or any product containing animal milk the night before, the sugar digestion will take much longer, and usually blood tests are done in the morning when there was still no time for the sugar crystals to be digested. The result of this exam is passed on to the doctor.

When poor digestion occurs, the intestine and colon release toxins that cause interference in the process of eliminating feces, creating many more future complications.

(See later a chapter written by Dr. Vanessa Albuquerque on the research of milk and its effect on the human body.)

What Needs To Be Eliminated

What has to be eliminated,
cannot be left within us.

How is the colon affected, and what happens in the colon when there is poor digestion?

When a person goes to the bathroom to defecate, the feces come out, but some of the waste remains. When the person goes to the bathroom again, the body puts out the residues that were left, new residues remain, and so on.

If there is no good digestion of the basic protein in the diet, the body creates a kind of glue that goes into the blood and makes the red blood cells aggregate to each other, causing a failure of the red blood cells to receive the necessary amounts of oxygen. This glue needs to be expelled, and, as the body has the ability to clean itself, it also comes out in the feces. The problem is done. The feces residues that should only be leaning against the internal walls of the colon or rectum, waiting to be expelled, are glued. They ferment and create toxins that can get into the bloodstream.

This is easy to see in the analysis of living blood. They

are not feces in the blood. They are toxins created by feces. Unfortunately, although science is already well advanced knowing about 5,000 different types of bacteria, there are still more than 30,000 that we don't know the origin of, or whether they are good or harmful to the body. They are part of the transformations or mutations. Microorganisms, bacteria, and fungi are present in the transformation stage in our body because we are formed of microorganisms that transform, bacteria that transform, fungi that transform, and so on.

These transformations must occur through a normal process, maintaining health, as long as the internal environment is also healthy. But if the internal environment is not favorable to the changes, due to the lack of oxygen, the simple transformations that should be beneficial to health will cause mutations. The system will then have to streamline reserves that can combat and expel these mutations. This could possibly be the origin of the organic deficiencies that can cause diseases if there are not enough defenses to fight them, or if the Lymphatic System does not expel them. If there is oxygen, there can be no infection, no inflammation, no illness. For that, we breathe all the time. Otherwise, we would die immediately from lack of oxygen.

Normally people who die in fires do not burn to death, they are asphyxiated by the lack of oxygen. Remember: when we breathe, we fill our lungs with oxygen, and the heart pumps blood to the lungs. Red blood cells hit the lung wall, receive oxygen, and carry it throughout the body. But if the red blood cells are glued to each other by the glue created from the poor digestion of proteins, they will not receive the amount of oxygen needed by the body, making parts of the body vulnerable. The body may get sick. This does not cause immediate death because we have about 100 trillion red blood cells, and hundreds of thousands are born every second, and hundreds of thousands die. But life is definitely shortening. There have always been diseases, since the beginning of the world, but most of the diseases that are present today are caused by the mutations that occur in the body, often caused by products we use without knowing if they are really good for our organism.

Breast Cancer

Today, it has become almost fashionable for people to have breast cancer. When we, as older adults, were children, we never heard that a woman had breast cancer. Today, the number of people with breast cancer is immense.

Why do I say "people" instead of "women"? Simple. It is because men are also liable to get breast cancer. I have dealt with several male breast-cancer patients.

Most of the time, breast cancer is caused by the use of products that prevent the extraction of toxins from the body. Deodorant kills toxins when they leave the body through the armpits, but the so-called "antiperspirant" in almost all deodorants today does not allow toxins to leave the body. The antiperspirant causes toxins to be trapped in a quadrant of breast tissue, damaging areas that will become diseased, resulting in breast cancer.

Many people think it's gross to see an armpit moistened with sweat and begin using an antiperspirant to prevent it happening to them. The stain will not appear because the toxins that were supposed to leave there will be retained.

These pores exist for extraction, and we must let the toxins out through sweat. Some people say they do not sweat. It is possible, but in these cases the body has to maintain another alternative eliminatory system to extract these toxins, or the body has a metabolism that does not produce sweat. This does not mean that the person is sick. It is the metabolism of each person, as it is with color blindness. The person who does not distinguish colors does not mean that he is sick. Rather, he was born that way. *(Today, there are lenses on the market that allow color blind people to see colors.)*

There are many recommendations for women to have mammograms. My recommendation is that you try to educate yourself about the consequences of a mammogram. I could talk about the side effects caused by mammography, while giving it a deserving credit. I suggest listening to Doctor Lair Ribeiro* who explains it very well. Once they become aware of the side effects caused by mammography, they certainly won't do it.

---

*About Dr. Lair Ribeiro

Graduated in Medicine for over 45 years, cardiologist, master in cardiology from PUC-RIO, nutrologist by ABRAN and Brazilian Medical Association, Dr. Lair Ribeiro lived for 17 years in the United States, during which time he worked in three American universities: Harvard Medical School, Baylor College of Medicine, and Thomas Jefferson University. During this period, he also held the positions of chief medical officer at Merck Sharp & Dohme and chief executive officer, rising to vice president, at Ciba Corporation, now Novartis.

Author of more than 100 scientific papers published in indexed American medical journals, Dr. Lair Ribeiro has also published 38 books, 15 of them best sellers, 26 translated into other languages, available today in more than 40 countries.

For over 20 years, he has given lectures in several Brazilian cities, several countries in South America, Central America, North America, and Europe. He has trained more than 4,000 Brazilian physicians in the area of Nutritional Adequacy and Optimization of Homeostasis.

Testimony of Lara Gois

My name is Lara Gois. I am a journalist and presenter. I met morphologist Jimmy Albuquerque in 2012 through an aunt who herself went for a consultation.

My aunt Neuza knew I was not healthy, and she encouraged me. I pointed out to her that I had already made an appointment with a hematologist and had already had some tests for which I would have the results soon. But, thank God, my aunt insisted, and I was able to make an appointment!

On my way to the appointment, I almost passed out driving as I passed over an overpass in St. Paul. I stopped the car, prayed and asked God for a chance. I called my pastor, Francisco, on the phone, and he told me that God had shown him that I had taken a test, during which my finger was pierced, like when they measure insulin!

I went to the appointment not knowing exactly what it was, and when Dr. Jimmy pierced my fingertip to test my blood, I remembered what the pastor had told me!

Dr. Jimmy told me that the discrepancies in my blood were many and that different diseases could develop. I almost fainted when driving because I didn't have enough oxygen. What survives in an organism with little oxygen? Cancer.

I decided to start that very day the diet, alkaline-based treatment and natural supplements that Dr. Jimmy suggested.

When I went to pick up the other blood tests, I opened the envelope already knowing what it was; the doctor told me I had two lymph nodes in my armpit and left breast, and she pointed me to the suggested conventional treatments. I told her that I would not do them, and she became very angry at my answer.

After 5½ months, I did the ultrasound and mammogram (last one, I haven't done it since). The tumors had disappeared. Seeing the results, the doctor asked me whether I had finally decided to follow the conventional protocol—chemotherapy, etc. I replied no, that I had done natural treatment with a renowned morphologist. She showed no interest in the course I had taken, despite the success I had. A great pity for her and her patients!

In addition to breast cancer, I had developed leukemia. Imagine all this together. But after 1 year and 4 months, my blood was completely clean and healthy.

I am very grateful to God for the life of Dr. Jimmy Albuquerque, one of the most amazing people I know. I am grateful to my aunt, who encouraged me to go to morphologist Jimmy; and I am grateful to everyone who referred him to her. That's why I always talk to people about my treatment, warn them that there are alternatives when traditional doctors tell you there are not. Maybe they don't know ... Then only God, and those who have been there before, can encourage you and give you direction!

I did my treatment in Brazil, and today I live in Europe, but I have always spread the news of this wonderful treatment and the work of this wonderful person who loves what he does.

Every treatment is a gift!

I try to help by organizing conferences in Europe, so that many more people know the technique of blood cleansing and can treat themselves as I have done.

I have also prepared an e-book that talks about the treatment. I have created useful recipes for the needed diet, and adapted others with the help of my grateful mother, Maria!

Today, I don't even know what it means to have the flu. I am always healthy. I eat normally. I am healed, and I advise everyone to take care of their health through blood treatment!

God bless you!
Lara Gois

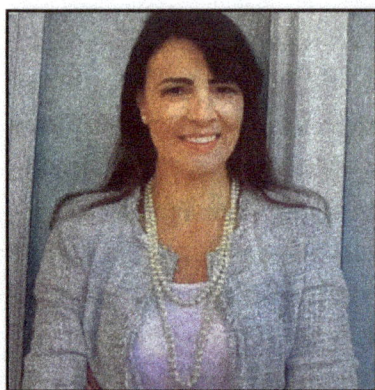

Lara Gois

Graduate in Journalism from
Universidade Nove de Julho

Specializing in Fashion, Lara Gois has participated in several television programs as a fashion and style consultant. Presenter graduated from Senac, worked for Nickelodeon as a children's presenter, commercial presenter in several Bstian stations. Actress graduated from Teatro Escola Macunaima, acted in several shows and TV programs, and record series. She has been modeling since she was 15 and still works in Brazil and Europe.

Writer of the e-book "Alkaline Food" and translator.

Facebook: Alimentação alcalina Lara Gois

https://www.facebook.com/lara.gois.52

Hippocrates, father of Western medicine, said:
For the patient to get the cure, it will be necessary
to give up the things that made him sick.

Effects Of Garlic
On The Body

Some time ago, I participated in lectures with Professor John Morton, successor of John Roger of the MSIA group (Movement of the Inner Path of the Soul). He explained that there could be no garlic in our diet. That made me feel a little confused at first because I always heard that garlic was good for health.

I decided to do some research and analyze the blood of people who had chronic illnesses, such as diseases in the esophagus, ulcers, constant heartburn, constant headaches, thyroid problems, itching, kidney infection, candidiasis, and even people with emotional problems. All were consumers of excess garlic. I started to suggest, along with cleaning the blood, that they stop the excessive consumption of garlic, and the result was incredible. All had almost immediate improvements.

The accumulated toxins that came out with the cleaning of the blood, and the absence of their consumption of garlic made these people healthy, without the physical and emotional disturbances they had before.

I saw a distinguished lady with several health problems. Her body gave off the smell of garlic. I suggested that she stop the excessive garlic consumption. I informed her that nothing in excess was good for the body and that every-thing in life must be in balance. She understood, and about four months later, she came to see me again, with another countenance.

She was like someone else, without the problems she had previously. She had cleaned the blood and stopped the consumption of garlic completely.

I would like to add a parenthesis here about garlic and how our body has the capacity to adapt. If you eat garlic and do not have different reactions in your body, such as itching, nausea, dizziness, headaches, etc., and you do not belch the taste of garlic when you eat, feel free to enjoy.

What needs to be expelled has to be expelled.
It cannot, and must not, stay within us.

Some Child Sicknesses

Another detail that I got in my research was in cases of sick children, where doctors did not discover the reason for the illnesses.

The mothers brought their children for me to do the blood analysis. We must remember that all the cells in our body work according to the vibrations of our thoughts, and that the child, the fetus, is directly connected to the mother before birth. I decided to ask the mothers if, when they got pregnant, they accepted the pregnancy normally, or if they had rejection of the newly formed fetus in their wombs. Some lied saying no, they did not have a pregnancy rejection. Why do I say they lied? Simply because some time later, they returned, confessing the problems they had during pregnancy. In almost all cases, there was a rejection by the mother.

Most were cases of total rejection. But for "other" reasons, they went through with the pregnancy. In these cases, the spiritual factor is important. I suggest to the mothers that they ask the child for forgiveness, and pray to God to give the son or daughter the power to heal. This has helped a lot so that these children can heal. I would like to make a reservation about the case of sick children. This information refers to the cases that were confirmed to me by mothers who rejected their children during pregnancy, but that does not mean that all childhood illnesses are caused by *in utero* rejection.

I pray because I believe in the power of prayer.

Speaking of body, it is good to give a brief explanation. But first I want to highlight one of the major disorders notified to patients by doctors.

Blood Pressure

You go to the doctor, and your blood pressure is measured, as well as your weight. For example, when the doctor measured your pressure, it was 150 over 90 (or 15x9). Regardless of whether the person really has a pressure problem, the emotional aspect of the moment may already have increased the pressure, or the barometric variation may also be high. Then the doctor says you have a problem and will be prescribed blood pressure medicine that you will have to take for the rest of your life. You have now become a dependent on the Pharmacy. But the doctor did not check the barometric pressure (of the atmospheric air) at the time he took your pressure, so he will not know if your body is balancing the atmospheric pressure. This is important because our body must always be in balance with the air pressure. Life is balance.

Aristotle stated that "Virtus in medium"— "Virtue is in the middle," or "Virtue is the art of finding the medium between the extremes."

Our body, being healthy, will be balancing its own pressure according to the pressure of the atmospheric air. I give as an example my blood pressure, which has always been stable at 14x8.5 (140x85) (this is my metabolism). There are people with metabolism whose pressures are low. But if the barometric pressure is above normal, my body will certainly increase my pressure to maintain balance, and it has already reached 17x 9 (170x90) a few times, which does not mean that I have a pressure problem.

Sometimes when I find through checking the meteorological service that the air pressure is high, and I check my pressure, there it is, above my normal: 14x8.5 (140x85). Another easy example to prove is that when a diver is under water, his pressure can reach very high numbers reaching 50 x10. This does not mean that the diver has pressure problems, but that the body is healthy by balancing the pressure around it, so much so that he, the diver, being in the depths cannot emerge immediately. You need to stop so that the body gradually decreases its own pressure, balancing each variation. Otherwise, you will have an embolism and may bleed from your ears and even your eyes, and the pain is horrible. For this purpose, there are decompression chambers, more commonly found in the Navy health departments, for emergencies in case the diver needs to emerge immediately.

In Brazil, some years ago, there were scales in pharmacies that for use, you would buy a card from the cashier, get on the machine that gave you written on a piece of paper, your blood pressure, your weight, your height. But it also gave information for which the reason was unknown to the people, which was the barometric pressure of the air at that moment. That information showed that if your blood pressure was high, the barometric pressure was possibly high. And in that case, he had no reason to worry because his body was balancing pressures. These scales are no more. They were available for about three years in pharmacies but were withdrawn because the people should not know the truth about blood pressure. I don't know if they have already heard that the pharmaceutical laboratory medical advice is determining that the pressure now needs to be low 10x7 (100x70).

If your blood pressure is above what they determine is normal, you will have to take blood pressure medicine for the rest of your life. This explanation does not mean that there are no people who really do have problems with high or low blood pressure.

I think the best medicine for pressure is in the Bible, where Paul says to Timothy:

"Your health problem is because you don't drink wine."

Although Timothy's problem was not one of pressure, wine does balance the pressure. I have already made this recommendation to several people who had pressure problems, and the improvement was immediate, including with Pastors who considered drinking wine a sin. If so, they would be sinners today because they were able to improve the pressure and stop taking the suggested remedies. Drinking wine to regulate the pressure does not mean getting drunk. My suggestion is that a cup of dry red wine espresso twice in the week before dinner is sufficient. But if you are going to drink the wine, buy a good, expensive wine. No drinking low or excess quality wines. For people who may have problems with wine rejection, they should not take it. Have you ever heard that a Pope, a Cardinal, or a Father had pressure problems? I think not! If you really have a pressure problem, it is because you are already sick for other reasons. And then, if wine was bad, I think Jesus Christ would have turned the water into orange juice.

Body Functions

We have a gland in our body called the TIMO Gland, responsible for the creation of leukocytes, which are white blood cells, associated with the immune and lymphatic systems. The production of hormones created by them is responsible for the general growth, mainly in the beginning of life that does the purifying work of defense of the body with the creation of white cells that attack elements harmful to the body, which are considered invaders to our organism. The "T" cells that are ordered to be created by the Thymus gland, are responsible for regulating our immune system. They are intelligent and work for our physiological needs, making themselves present whenever necessary. But it is necessary to remember

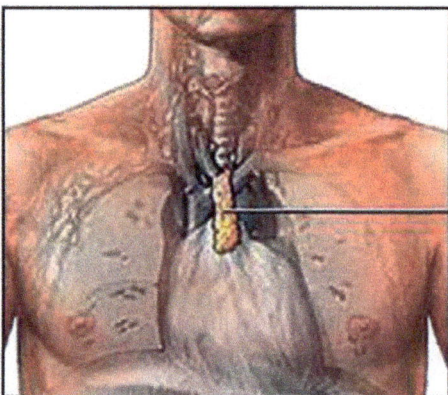

Thymus

that for the body, through the Timo gland, to develop a healthy system, it will be necessary that there are the basic elements that contribute to this existence, which is and will always be digested food.

Few professionals know or talk about the side effects caused by chemotherapy or radiotherapy in Timo, which will stop organizing to produce the leukocytes needed for healing. In order for us to have a better view of the importance of Timo, if a child is born without the thymus, it will have poor heart formation, a series of psychiatric problems, mental retardation, growth deficiency, facial deformity, cognitive behaviors, and a poor immune behavior, causing the life span too be shortened. Scientists have already proven that in autoimmune diseases, the immune system attacks its own proteins, mistaking them for foreign bodies. This is certainly caused by poor digestion, which did not properly form or transform the protein. Looking at this aspect, the protein passed to really be a different element within us.

Obviously, we cannot fail to emphasize the emotional factor that has a direct influence on the digestion and metabolization of food. As all the cells in our body work according to the vibrations created by our thoughts, if we worry or get bored, especially at meal times, there will be no good digestion. The time for the meal should be in complete harmony. One of the pleasures of life is to eat, so why not make that a moment of real pleasure? Forget the worries, the adversities. Turn off, live the moment of meals with total pleasure, not like an obligation to stay alive.

We Eat More
Than We Need

We usually eat more than is necessary. I did a test one time with a young man who worked in construction. I was in a Brazilian restaurant in Florida, and I saw that this guy, who sat at the table next to me, had a plate with a lot of food. The amount he had on the plate would have fed me about three times. I asked if he always ate a lot that way, and he answered me saying that he needed it and that he was very hungry because he worked hard and needed a lot of food. I made him a proposal: I would pay for his lunch for a week if he agreed to eat for a day as I eat. He asked me how it would be, and I replied that I would eat the same thing as him. He agreed, and we set the day. We arrived at the restaurant and went to the queue to do our dishes because it was self-service food by the kilo. He was filling his plate, and I was right behind behind choosing the food he put on his plate, only I put a lot less than he did. We went for weighing, and the cost of his food was very high. My dish had much less food, so the cost was much lower.

We sat down at the table, and I told him he could start. He put a huge mouthful in his mouth and then a bigger one. Then I said, "Now you will imitate me." I put a small amount of food on the fork and brought it to my mouth, starting to chew. I did not give the 32 chews suggested for optimal digestion, but I got about 20 chews and swallowed. He looked at me, and I said, "Now eat like I did, slowly." It was even fun for both of us to eat. As I had little food, I finished faster, while his plate was still full.

As soon as I was done, I told him to keep eating. He ingested a few more mouthfuls and started saying that he had lost his hunger. At this point, I explained that he had lost his hunger because his body was satisfied. Now that he had chewed his food well, he had satisfied the glands in his mouth that determined what the body really needed.

Hunger was not in the stomach. The stomach could ask for food. It was the glands in the mouth that had to be satisfied that would determine the right amount for the body. As he ate fast almost without chewing, his stomach was getting full, but if he satisfied the glands in his mouth, he would not need to eat that much. He laughed and said, "Now I'm going to save on my food." I laughed, too. I haven't seen him in a long time, but I think he had an experience that could be enjoyed for the rest of his life.

Since I spoke in excess, I now go with my point of view, to contradict the teachings that many had. I will talk about the excess water.

Excessive Water Damages The Body

once gave a lecture to a group of elderly people in Brasilia and decided to ask about the water consumption of each person present. To my surprise, most of the people over 90 did not drink more than a glass of water a day, and most forgot to drink.

The question is: If doctors say that we need to drink more than a liter of water a day, why didn't those old people drink a lot of water? Some informative theories launched through scientific positions were that the elderly person's body does not need a lot of liquid, so he does not drink much water. But in my research, I found that these same elderly people were never adept at drinking a lot of water, even when they were younger.

My mother, who passed away at the age of ninety, said that she only drank water when she was thirsty. If the rule that we need to drink a lot of water is general for everyone, why don't these older people fit this rule?

During the five years that I lived on the West Coast of Africa, I interacted with many old people, including a distinguished lady known as Mama Martins, one of the last Brazilian slaves to return to Nigeria, where her family became rich with the introduction of artesian wells and selling water to the local natives. At the time, she was 105 years old. I asked her if, since the family sold water, she should drink enough water to maintain her health and vigor. Another knowledge was acquired that day when she said that she only drank water when she was thirsty and never more than a cup.

So I decided to read a little bit about how the camel fills his belly, so he can cross immense distances in the desert. The camel is large and certainly needs water to survive. However, camels do not use all the water stored in their belly. They consume a little at a time so they can reach their destinations. The daily consumption of the camel is negligible, considering its size.

Today, after my cure, without drinking a lot of water and having done more than 5,000 analyses of live blood, where I see that people who drink a lot of water have blood aggregation caused by poor digestion of the protein, I bring in my memory this episode of that lady of 105 years old who only drank when she was thirsty, which confirms that we must obey our bodies' need, but not always what they tell us to do. Let us consider that diseases proliferate because of poor digestion. So we need to pay attention to the detail of these oral enzymes being constantly washed out of our mouth, esophagus, and stomach with excess water ingested.

These enzymes are responsible for the digestion of food: protein, fat, and sugar. I attended several athletes whose diet was perfect and who drank more water than necessary, whose blood showed poor protein digestion. Wity a simple recommendation for them to drink if they were thirsty, the blood had already normalized in a few days. What I have noticed is that most people are addicted to water. I once saw an athlete who came to see me because he was constantly tired without reason, even though he had a perfect diet. He now understood why his body was getting tired. I asked him if he drank a lot of water, and the answer was emphatic: it is because they said I need to drink a lot of water. So, I said to him that this can be addiction. He immediately objected, saying that he drank a lot of water because he liked water. I was forced to clarify that those who use cocaine use it because they like it, those who use marijuana use it because they like it, whoever uses drugs does it because they like it. Isn't this excess when you feed an addiction?

He decided to make a personal experience and reduced the amount of water ingested. He started drinking only when his body asked for it, and the result was surprising. He acquired more resistance. I constantly see information on the internet, on television, and even in the written media, saying that we need to drink a lot of water. Most of the sick people with cancer that I have seen used to drink a lot of water. All, without exception, were indoctrinated to drink a lot of water. My recommendation is that you obey the body.

If your body needs fluid,
it makes you thirsty: DRINK!

If your body needs food,
it makes you feel hungry: EAT!

If your body needs rest,
it makes you feel tired: REST!

"Once again: It is the body that dictates
the rules of the game, and nothing
in excess is good for the body."

Another detail about water consumption is that I constantly see people suggesting drinking a glass of water in the morning before breakfast, and some even suggest adding lemon. It may have some benefit, but it will certainly wash away the oral enzymes necessary for digestion. When my illness started, it was suggested to me to drink a glass of water with lemon every day. I did this for a long time, and my illness was gaining ground within me. When I found out that I needed the oral enzymes in order to have a good digestion, I stopped completely, and the results were great. The cure came more and more each day. That is why I wrote this book, which must disagree with things that are transmitted to us daily through the media. In order to clean the blood and have the red cells receiving and transmitting oxygen in the body, constant digestion is necessary. But for that, we need the oral enzymes constantly available to perform the task of digestion.

During the night, we accumulate enzymes in our mouth, esophagus, and inlet valve in the stomach, which closes when food enters so that we don't have reflux. Oral enzymes are necessary for the digestion of protein, fat, and sugar foods (mentioned previously) that are added to stomach acids for digestion of food that is then transformed into feces.

When we drink the water on an empty stomach, we wash away these enzymes, and the digestion will certainly not be the same. If our body was created to produce these enzymes for digestion, why do we destroy them with oral hygiene products that kill the enzymes? This is not to mention that we wash them away when we ingest fasting water, washing them from the mouth, esophagus, and valve entering the stomach and not allowing them to do their job. I suggest taking enzymes to almost all the people with whom I do the blood analysis when I find the glued cells due to poor digestion of the protein, so that they have a better digestion.

When they return for the second blood test, and the cells are still glued together, I am aware that these people drink water while fasting, especially with lemon. I suggest that they temporarily stop the fasting water consumption and ask them to return after a few days for a new blood analysis. The result is always the same: The red cells have totally detached from each other and are carrying oxygen to the body. In other words, they have perfect protein digestion.

The information contained here is part of my experience for my own healing and the healing of all those people who followed my therapy and were cured.

Diseases Caused By Bad Food Digestion

*L*et's see in this table what can cause bad digestion of each of the three foods:

PROTEINS • FAT • SUGAR

PROTEIN	FAT	SUGAR
URATE CRYSTALS MONOSODIUM	WASTE FROM WASTE FOOD CONSTANTS	SUGAR CRYSTALS
FORMATION OF URIC ACID	PLATES OF FAT PLATES	FUNGI FROM YEASTS
KIDNEY STONES	HARDENING OF THE ARTERIES	CANDIDA
ENRICHMENTS OF THE MUSCLES	HIGH PRESSURE	SPILLS AND DIABETES
ARTHRITIS	STROKE	LOW IMMUNITY
CARDIAC DISEASES	CARDIAC DISEASES	CARDIAC DISEASES

Human Death Starts With The Cell That Produces Human Life Also

Excerpted from biomedical criticism
Compiled by Doctor Richard Murray

The human body is made up of (between) 80 and 100 trillion cells. Approximately 1 billion cells per hour must be replaced … 24 billion cells per day, which require all known elements of nutrition. Each of the 100 trillion cells in the human body contains 300 to 800 cell components in each of the cell energy sources, cells called mitochondria. Each mitochondria in the liver cells contains about 5,000 respiratory units, while mitochondria in the heart cells have up to 20,000 respiratory units. And about 30 trillion red blood cells circulate through 70,000 km of blood vessels. A normal healthy person produces 15 million red blood cells per second.

Autopsies have shown that people who eat mostly cooked food will have their pancreas dangerously enlarged with malfunction, often on the verge of collapse. If the pancreas is forced, day after day, year after year, to produce an excess of digestive enzymes, the rest of the body's enzyme reserve is severely affected. Most young people do not seem to suffer from the negative effects of this overload.

Anatomy of A Cell

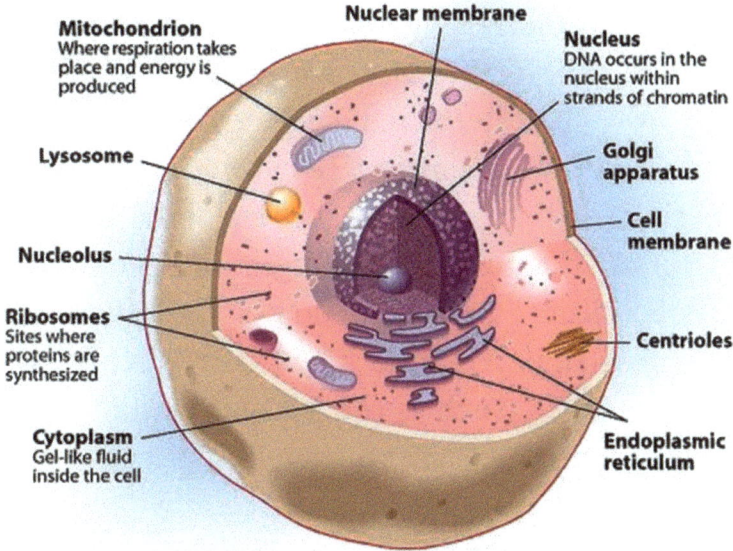

Mitochondrion
Where respiration takes
place and energy is
produced

Nuclear membrane

Nucleus
DNA occurs in the
nucleus within
strands of chromatin

Lysosome

**Golgi
apparatus**

**Cell
membrane**

Nucleolus

Ribosomes
Sites where
proteins are
synthesized

Centrioles

Cytoplasm
Gel-like fluid
inside the cell

**Endoplasmic
reticulum**

Red Globulus

Gradually, the overloaded pancreas and other digestive organs will not be able to produce sufficient amounts of endogenous metabolic enzymes. This leads to digestive diseases and toxic intestinal conditions. According to Doctor Edward Howell in his book, *Enzyme Nutrition,* in the enzymatic concept, a pancreas that is not working well is related to the increase of chronic degenerative diseases and cancer. And, in this case, death begins in the colon. Enzymes and fibers are essential for proper digestion and elimination. Unfortunately, the typical American diet is significantly lacking in such requirements. Fiber acts as an agent of volume, transit time, and the speed of food in the digestive tract. These actions are to prevent metabolic waste that create toxic byproducts.

A major advantage of fiber is that it binds bile acids and carries bile, along with excess fats, out of the body. Fiber helps to lower cholesterol, reduce the risk of heart disease, lower blood pressure, improves blood sugar level, and promotes the growth of friendly intestinal flora. It also promotes intestinal regularity, aids digestion and helps keep the intestine clean. Fiber cannot do its job effectively unless enzymes do theirs. Over time, it becomes difficult to digest protein-rich foods (such as cooked meat and others deficient in food enzymes) that deplete the digestive organs, until they can no longer function efficiently.

This results in the accumulation of partially digested food in the intestine. In middle age, many people have up to 20 pounds of undigested, putrefactive food in their colon. (!!) Toxins produced from this putrefying buildup are reabsorbed into the bloodstream, creating autointoxication or self-poisoning resulting in a dramatically weakened immune system and can lead to serious debilitating health problems including colon cancer. Colon cancer is the most prevalent cancer in the world. Supplemental food enzymes taken with meals and between meals can work to help eliminate the accumulation of toxic waste in the stomach and colon.

Enzymes act as catalysts for foreign substances throughout the body preventing joint problems to prevent arteries from clogging. Enzymes in blood cells are responsible for the destruction of foreign bodies, substances that produce substances in the blood and lymph. During illness and infection, white blood cells increase to fight pathogens. When cooked food is digested, the body reacts as if we have an acute illness. Within 30 minutes of eating cooked food, our white blood cell count increases dramatically. This means that the immune system is being put into action unnecessarily, almost every time we eat.

Studies show that the mobilization and increase of white blood cells does not happen when raw food is consumed. The molecules of improperly digested proteins and fats are small enough to enter the blood, but too large to enter cells. They are called immune complex floats. They are now considered toxic invaders in the body instead of nutrients. It is very important to know the physiological divisions of the stomach. In the pyloric: chyme liquid accumulates here and drips into the duodenum. In the duodenum: enzymes of animal origin only work here because they do not work in the stomach, they do not save the energy of the digestive body, and the pancreas still produces identical enzymes. Basically: Food enzymes work here. In the body: hydrochloric acid and pepsin work here.

**Without good digestion, we will not die
of old age. Life will just shorten.**

The Stomach

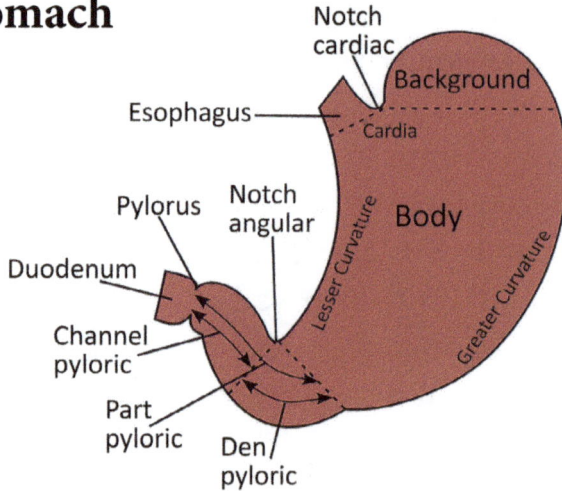

Previously, when I referred to the internal environment as being favorable (oxygenation), I meant that all digested food will be transformed, and what is no longer needed by the body will be extracted by normal delivery processes. But if the internal environment is not favorable (total oxygenation), our body will not make the transformation, but mutations will occur. Our body was not created for mutations, but for transformations.

The Importance Of
Live Blood Analysis

I am not the pioneer in the analysis of living blood. That has been known for many years. But I am a pioneer in curing cancer with my blood cleaning therapy because that is what cured me of a deadly cancer (Glio Blastoma Multiforme grade 4). No one had ever before been healed from this cancer.

Dr. Vanessa Albuquerque, a bio-medical doctor, and my student in the Morphology course (study of living blood), made a very good dissertation on the analysis of living blood, which I will review for you here:

The analysis of living blood, although it was the evolutionary beginnings of discoveries from blood that caused reagents to be created, facilitating the work of laboratory technicians and with that the analysis of live blood was practically forgotten because laboratories research to discover disease, not what causes disease. Obviously, they will find, through reagents, many discrepancies, deficiencies, and anomalies, as well as necessary elements for the body in its normal state, leading to a reading, but that through the analysis of live blood, in these possible readings made in the laboratory, the causes of the diseases do not appear, only illnesses alone.

Of course, laboratories can also find out if the body is deficient in white blood cells, reduced red blood cells, increased cholesterol, platelets, etc. I would like to cite an example of the analysis of live blood and its results:

Approximately 4 years ago, I did a friend's blood analysis. I noticed that he was not digesting protein because the RBCs (red cells) were all glued together (when we don't digest the protein, we create a kind of glue in the plasma, which is the water of the blood, causing the red cells to add to each other). This prevents red blood cells, red cells, or many also called red blood cells, from doing their job of receiving and transmitting oxygen to the body.

When we breathe and fill the lungs with oxygen, the heart pumps blood to the lungs. If the red cells, the erythrocytes, are separated and healthy when they hit the walls of the lungs, they receive oxygen and leave, distributing oxygen to the whole body. But if they are glued because of the poor digestion of proteins, they cannot receive or transmit the necessary oxygen to the rest of the body. This is the beginning of any illness, and it has been the most common one.

Alzheimer's, Parkinson's, and dementia are caused by a lack of oxygen in the brain, which gradually causes atrophy of the internal tissues. This will cause damage that is often irreparable. Considering that 20% of the oxygen that we acquire through breathing, food, and water goes to the brain through red blood cells, I notified my friend that he was not receiving the necessary amount of oxygen in his brain, and this could cause a disturbance in the brain that could cause an illness like Alzheimer's or even Parkinson's.

Approximately four years after I had his blood tested, I was called to his home and saw that he already had Parkinson's disease because his right hand was shaking a lot. I asked him if he had cleaned his blood as I had suggested, and he said no because the doctor said that what I had found in his blood would not cause illness. He showed me the tests done in laboratories. It was not surprising to me that because his lab tests were perfect, there was nothing unusual. He asked, "Why am I sick then if my exams show everything perfect?" I explained to him that for a long time, his brain was being damaged from lack of oxygen. This could cause a possible illness to develop, such as 100% Alzheimer's or Parkinson's. Although, trying to disqualify the work, many doctors criticize the morphology that is the study of living blood.

I want to make it very clear that it was through the analysis of living blood that I discovered the cause of the disease that formed in my own body: GBM (Glio Blastoma Multiforme grade 4). With this discovery, I worked to cleanse my blood. I also considered a Bible verse written about 1785 years before Christ that says:

"The life of the flesh is in the blood" (Leviticus 17:11).

Since the life of the flesh is in the blood, why not cleanse the blood?

And today, cured for more than 9 years, I closed my four companies in the United States to dedicate myself to health, helping people to understand that *if the blood is clean, there is no disease left in the body.*

This statement is very simple. When you go to the doctor, what does he ask for immediately? A blood test done in laboratories. He can also ask to have a stool or urine sample, or an MRI scan, etc. But the main thing they will never stop asking for is blood. It is because they know that blood carries life. However, it also carries death if it is dirty. The analysis of living blood shows what is really going on in the body because the blood is still alive. We can find many divergences, anomalies resulting from poor digestion.

We even find food residues not yet consumed by the body or that bile has not done its job of eliminating, those residues that continue to feed the body. If there is an anomaly in the production of bile, an unnecessary addition of bile, there will be marked thinness, where the body will be using all its physical reserves. This does not mean that the person is sick. It is a matter of the metabolism of each person. The body seeks adaptation. But if the production of bile is totally deficient, these food residues will remain in the blood feeding the body for a long time, causing obesity.

Many doctors and experts in the human body will say that it is a matter of hormones, possibly hormones that are missing or are in excess and impairing the work of other organs. Yes, it can be, but for sure, it is because of poor digestion constantly causing organic disturbances in the excessive or diminished production of these hormones. (Look at the graph of the dominoes.) This anomaly in digestion can even cause anemia. There are obese people who discover in laboratory tests that they are anemic. Why then? Why are there both fat and anemic people? Anemia is not a disease. It is a sign of a series of disorders caused in the body.

We therefore have to find out which organic factors are not in perfect working order. This is what the analysis of living blood is for, to show whether a person digests the three basic foods:

Sugar • Fat • Protein

Animal Milk

Many people ask me to explain why milk is banned from my list of acidic and alkaline foods.

Dr. Vanessa Albuquerque did a survey regarding the results of ingesting animal milk in our body. I transcribe her material with pleasure.

The body's need related to the consumption of cow's milk can be understood as a myth fueled by the beliefs issued by the industries marketing milk as an essential food for maintaining health and a source of calcium for bones. However, studies show the opposite, characterizing the end of innocence in relation to the myth that "milk is good for health," which remained rooted as a cultural phenomenon for a long time. This lead the human body to acquire innumerable inflammatory processes, which can start from a simple cold to more serious pathologies like cancer.

MILK INGESTION MAKES FRAGILE BONES

The human body is intelligent in all its functioning, and for this reason there is a natural tendency to create stages of compensation when we place on it some type of demand capable of impairing its performance. Milk, because it contains large proteins for human metabolism, acidifies the environment during the digestion process, leading the body's need to use the calcium present in the body as an acid neutralizer and when unbalancing the Ph (hydrogen potential), calcium loss occurs on the bones. Because the calcium stored in the bones is released to compensate for the excessive acidity in the body. Over time, the bones become brittle. Some studies show that in countries where people consume more dairy products there is a higher incidence of osteoporosis. In addition to not providing the calcium the body needs, milk works by releasing the body's important calcium to the bones.

Milk Pasteurization Increases Obesity Indices

The nutritional properties of milk are destroyed by going through the pasteurization process, in which heat is able to eliminate enzymes, including phosphatase that is an essential enzyme for calcium absorption. In addition to pasteurization, antibiotics, hormones, and other medications are added to milk. Therefore, the final consumer not only drinks milk without nutritional properties but also without all the possible elements that can be used by the body.

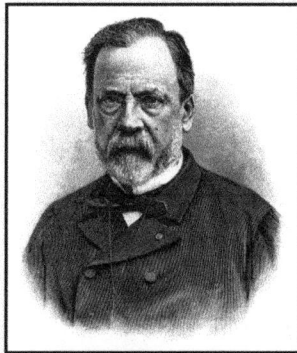

Louis Pasteur, although Béchamp's plagiarist, was against pasteurization of milk.

Low-fat products became very popular when obesity reached epidemic proportions. However, in the case of low-fat milk, as soon as the fat is removed, it is replaced by sugars that can potentially be more harmful than the whole product. The US Department of Agriculture (USDA) and the American Academy of Pediatrics have formulated guidelines for people to limit consumption of sugar-sweetened beverages, but this recommendation has not extended to low-fat milk. That is, cow's milk is ideal for calves. Milk of one's own species is suitable for babies of the same species, so cow's milk is ideal for consumption by calves. (That is, animal milk is for its own offspring.) We are the only species (besides the birds that domesticated) that drinks milk after childhood, milk of a different species. When childhood ends around the age of four, it may occur that we stop producing lactase, the enzyme responsible for breaking down lactose in milk and dairy products.

Diseases And The Evils Caused By Milk Consumption

Ingestion of milk by an organism that does not produce lactase can result in abdominal cramps, gas, nausea, bloating and diarrhea, anemia, childhood diabetes, heart disease, kidney stones, malnutrition, various inflammations, infertility in women, osteoporosis, atherosclerosis, and many other problems. Even in the case of individuals who continue to produce lactase after adulthood, they will not benefit from drinking milk, as our body was not created to digest milk. Even those who do not have an intolerance have consequences when ingesting it. Milk is mucus-forming, which makes its consumption harmful, even in the case of a simple cold, and contributes to respiratory problems and allergies of all kinds. Scientist **Richard Panush,** in a study with rabbits, did the experiment to "produce" inflamed joints in animals just by replacing water with milk.

In another study, scientists observed more than 50% reduction in arthritis pain when participants eliminated milk and dairy products from their diet. Most milk is homogenized, which denatures proteins, making it even more difficult to digest. Many people react to these proteins as if they were foreign bodies causing an overreaction in the immune system. Studies have also linked homogenized milk to heart disease. According to **José Saramago**, the text is incisive when referring to the custom of consuming milk and dairy products: "Using the metaphor of *The Essay on Blindness*, we can imagine milk consumption as a custom followed by everyone, in a kind of blindness that affects us, and it is contagious, leading us to go through painful experiences, until our mental and moral autonomy in the matter of diet are reestablished."

We think that if a fresh food is sold, then it does not contain poisonous ingredients. This is a mistake we make. But most of us discover that he lived eating. If it were for the balance of the metabolism of the body itself, he should not have eaten, when he receives confirmation that he has cancer, diabetes, allergies, arthritis, hypercholesterolemia, obesity, steatosis, renal or biliary lithiasis, atherosclerosis, Parkinson's disease (milk sickness), etc.

The myth that milk is necessary and pure is dispelled. Every food we eat should have the three basic foods—protein, sugar, and fat. When we eat foods that have had the fat removed, the body is being deprived of fat, which is a nutrient needed to stay healthy. In this case, as we eat foods without fat, the body will tend to retain as much fat as possible, possibly generating obesity. Yeah! … No animal drinks milk after it is grown up. Only us, and the others. Neither is meant for us! …

Hemotherapy[5]

When we analyze people's blood, we discover the absence or excess of red blood cells or white blood cells, sugar crystals, and uric acid crystals. But when we see that there is a deficiency of white blood cells in the blood, we need to recommend to the person who has this deficiency to undergo Hemotherapy[5]. Any and all healing will only occur if there are defenses, leukocytes, which are white blood cells. These recommendations are based on the more than proven effect created in the transport of blood from the vein to the muscle (arm or gluteal region). The body creates defense in 24 hours. So that they can educate themselves more about hemotherapy, I suggest going online and listening to **Doctor Luís Moura,** who was one of the most successful doctors to have achieved hemotherapy in their patients. Although this process helps to create defenses, I want to make two things clear, especially to my therapist friends.

First: If a person has leukemia, he cannot do hemo-

---

5 **Review Note**

Hemotherapy - In medicine, the parenteral introduction of human blood (or parts thereof) for therapeutic purposes, either to replenish an anemic or exsanguinated Stras. fusion, or to implement a 'passive immunization'.

Source: http://www.treccani.it/enciclopedia/emoterapia/

therapy because this disease is already an excess of white blood cells. It is the cleaning of the blood that will bring the results against this disease.

Second: Never do ozone hemotherapy. Why? Simple! When the responsible person draws the patient's blood, every type of anomaly that is in the patient's blood comes into the syringe, such as fungi, toxins, germs, parasites, bacteria, and others. The moment that same blood is placed intramuscularly in the patient himself, the body immediately creates defenses to neutralize the foreign bodies that have now been injected back. But, as with oxygen, there is no infection or inflammation in the body. The moment the blood is added to ozone, or vice versa, all these anomalies that cause illness die. And hemotherapy will no longer have the effect for which it was intended because the body no longer needs to create defenses. A sacrifice with no positive result. Ozone can be made separately from hemotherapy with an interval of at least one day between them.

Urinotherapy[6]

A nother way to obtain similar results for the body to acquire more defenses is with urine therapy, very well explained by orthomolecular medicine in the world and in particular by the **Jesuit Father Renato Bartth of Cuiabá**. Rather persecuted by the pharmaceutical industry, he was even arrested. Urine therapy causes the body to receive the lost natural hormones, enzymes, and antibiotics, and does not allow harmful substances to enter the blood. However, the most important thing in urine therapy is that the body creates, as in hemotherapy, extra defenses to combat unwanted foreign bodies. See this note on urine therapy found on the internet *(next page)*:

---

6 **Review Note - Urine Therapy**

In the ancient Sanskrit text *Sri Damartantram* the use of urine is reported.

In **traditional Indian medicine**, urine is indicated to treat diseases of the elderly, eye ailments, coughs, digestive and hepatic problems. For external use it is recommended as a treatment for burns and wounds.

HISTORY

The history of urine therapy reports the use of urine by the Chinese and in ancient Greece. **Pliny** *(23-79 AD)*, **Galen** *(129-199) and* **Paracelsus** *(1493-1541)* mention this method.

In addition, in earlier times the observation of urine for diagnostic purposes played an important role; recall in this regard the Indian, Egyptian, Tibetan and Hippocratic medicines. It was in the West and in Germany that the use of urine for therapeutic purposes became widespread, and it was the physician **Paullini** *(1643-1712)*, author of the text *The Pharmacopoeia of Waste*, who explained the use of urine, with his famous motto "Urine is a short way to a long life." *Continued on next page*

"Although urine therapy has been used for millennia by Egyptians, Chinese, and Indians, there is still no scientific evidence that it is really effective." Of course! It will never be classified as scientific evidence. There is no gain for the pharmaceutical industry. There will only be scientific proof if there is profit for the pharmaceutical industry. Look at what the Nobel Prize in medicine Dr. Richard Roberts said: "Pharmaceuticals block medicines that cure because they are not profitable."

---

6 **Review Note - Urine Therapy** *Continued*
ADVANTAGES OF THE METHOD
Laurin therapy, also called **autourotherapy**, is definitely a natural method with numerous advantages such as:
it is simple
it does not cost anything
it is usable in all diseases
With need for medical examination and diagnosis, easy learning of the method, immediate availability, and use for first aid helican as first aid for snake and scorpion bites.
Urine used as a remedy has both **indicative** and **regulatory** function, no drug can have such a 'breadth of action.'
The most difficult problem to be solved, for those who decide to resort to such treatment, is that of overcoming prejudices, which condition with the idea that urine is both something unclean and repulsive.
Numerous urine therapy experts have tried to explain how urine intake can maintain or restore health status, reminding us that 'urine therapy works both **preventively** and in **acute** and **chronic** diseases.'
SOURCE: http://www.naturopatiaeuropea.it/index.php/indice-lettera-u/414-u-rhinotherapy

What The Nobel Medicine Award Says

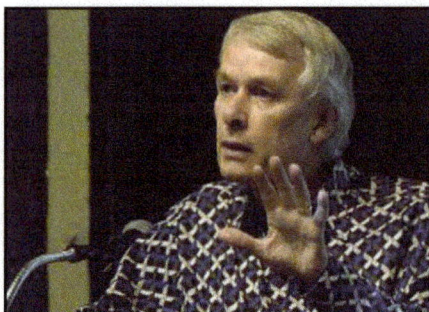

Dr. Richard J. Roberts

The Nobel Prize in Medicine winner, Richard J. Roberts, denounces the way large pharmaceutical companies work within the capitalist system, preferring economic benefits to health, and halting scientific progress in curing diseases because curing is not as profitable as chronic, long-lasting conditions. It has recently been revealed that major US pharmaceutical companies spend hundreds of millions of dollars a year on payments to doctors who promote their drugs. In addition, we reproduce this interview with Nobel Prize winner, Richard J. Roberts, who says that the drugs that cure are not profitable and therefore are not developed by pharmaceutical companies that, instead, develop drugs that are for long-lasting diseases or conditions. This, says Dr. Roberts, also prevents some drugs that could cure a disease from being investigated. Dr. Roberts also asks the question: *To what extent is it valid and ethical for the health industry to be governed by the same values and principles as the capitalist market?*

June 18, 2011
Originally published in La Vanguardia
Translation by Ana Bárbara Pedrosa

According to a publication in the **Journal of the American Medical Association**, the third leading cause of death in the United States is medical treatment. (For example: The person goes to the doctor, who gives treatment, and the person dies.) According to the **American Department of Health and Human Services** (in the United States), 15,000 people die each month, with medical treatment, in the United States. How many would this be in less developed countries?

(Information from Dr. Peter Glidden, B.S., N.D.)

Animals Teach

I like to use animals as examples of natural survival. Animals do not drink before eating, do not drink when they eat, and do not drink after they eat. They wait for digestion to happen, unless they have eaten some salty or spicy food. They know when they need to eat foods that help them to heal, or simply not to eat at all.

Consider the dog, for example. When he has some intestinal disorder, the first thing he eats is grass. Have you paid any attention to that? When the animal has a wound, he licks the wound to launch the oral bacteria in defense of possible foreign bodies that are already in the wound, or to prevent them from entering the body through it.

Every animal THINKS when it wakes up or stays in a state of inertia for a long time.

Newborn children also stretch. Have you noticed that? A simple stretch sends oxygen and energy to the nerves that were in a state of inertia. Let's see, for example, when we spend a lot of time in one position, sitting or even driving, when we get up, we feel a slight discomfort in the joints. For some, even pain is present. But if we stretch before we start walking, the discomfort disappears, and the pain even goes away.

I travel a lot by plane, often more than eight hours in flight. I constantly get up for a simple stretch. I have seen some airlines that encourage passengers to stretch out before starting disembarkation, especially on long journeys.

CHILDREN ALSO TEACH

As I said about the children previously, I would like to highlight some details because, as adults, we need to pay more attention to children. Children are born, they stretch, and after a few months, they start to crawl. Everyone thinks it's beautiful, and it is.

Then they try to stand! This is when the parents, or the grandparents, come and scream: *"Hold it so it doesn't fall!"* Let it fall! If a child does not try to stand, he will never walk. This is divine creation.

We Need To Risk

Risk is necessary to obtain results, other than the ones we already have. Those who do not have the capacity to take risks will normally be stagnant in time, without progress. But this is caused by fear, which is the worst feeling and the enemy of human beings. Life is risk. The person who does not risk does nothing, achieves nothing, and is a "John Nobody."[7] You can avoid some loss by not risking, but for sure:

- You can only love if you risk exposing your love.
- You can only laugh if you risk looking like a fool.
- You can only get involved if you risk contacting.
- You can only express your feelings when you expose yourself.
- You can only have a full life if you risk having it.
- You can only win if you risk investing.
- You can only see if you risk looking.

---

7 **Review Note**

John Doe is a name usually used in U.S. legal jargon to refer to a man whose real identity is unknown or is to be kept as such. This appellation was allegedly first used in the time of Edward the 1st of England during a legal diatribe called the Acts of Ejectment, in which, for convenience, a hypothetical landowner was referred to by the invented name John Doe. In time the expression began to be used to refer to a person whose identity is unknown, such as in the case of the discovery of an unidentified corpse until it is recognized. In Italy it is the equivalent of Ignoto or NN (from the Latin *nomen nescio*).

- You can only feel if you risk touching.
- You can only drive if you risk learning.
- Only those who have the ability to risk are free.
- In life, everything is a risk: The world is in the hands of those who have the capacity to dream and run the risk of living their dreams.

Risks need to be made.

Small risks encourage greater risks for great achievements. Only those who risk can succeed. The successful ones took a risk, even though they knew they could fail. Not everyone who tried succeeded, but certainly everyone who succeeded tried. If you have the ability to risk, you have already achieved 50% of success, but if you do not have this capacity, you have already obtained 100% of failure.

In Matthew 13:12, it is said that: *He who has will be given more. But for those who don't have it, it will be taken away* (paraphrased).[8] But to have it, you will have to risk getting it. In Mark 11:23, he says: *All things are possible for the one who believes.*

---

8 **Review Note**—THE PARABLE OF THE TALENTS. MATTHEW 25:24-30.

24 Then the one who had received only one talent also approached, and said: "Lord, I knew that thou art a hard man, reaping where thou hast not sown and gathering where thou hast not scattered; 25 I was afraid and went and hid thy talent under the ground; here is thine." 26 His master answered him, "Wicked servant and slacker, you knew that I reap where I did not sow and reap where I did not scatter; 27 you should therefore have taken my money to the bankers: when I returned I would have withdrawn mine with interest. 28 Therefore take away his talent, and give it to him who has the ten talents. 29 For to everyone who has, it shall be given, and he shall overflow; but to him who has not, even what he has shall be taken away. 30 And that worthless servant, cast him into the darkness outside. There shall be weeping and the gnashing of teeth."

During the period in which I was sick, I was risking all treatments, without positive results. I continued to risk it until I was successful in getting my cure. This was a risk where all attempts had failed. Edison, the creator of the electric lamp, when asked if he was not frustrated with so many attempts he had made, replied that every time he made a mistake, he knew he was wrong, that it was not that way, and he tried otherwise. The positive result comes from the determination in relation to the purpose, to the objective because only the determined ones are successful. Determine your future. Work to get where you want to go.

If you determine that you want to go to Paris next year, but right now you don't even have a job, don't worry. Work for your purpose with determination because God sends resources anyway, especially to the determined ones.

I would like to explain a little about depression, but for that I need to talk about a conversation with God. He, God, speaks to us through thoughts. God once told me that He needed to tell me something that I had never heard from any pastor, priest, rabbi, or any holy father in life. He told me that He speaks any language, but that He only speaks one word in whatever language He speaks.

I asked: *What word is that, God?* And He said to me: *The word is "YES."*

- *If you want to be happy, I say "yes."*
- *If you want to be sad, I say "yes."*

- *If you want to be optimistic, I say "yes."*
- *If you want to be pessimistic, I say "yes."*
- *If you want to be good, I say "yes."*
- *If you want to be bad, I say "yes."*
- *If you want to be an entrepreneur, I say "yes."*
- *If you want to be what nothing does in life, I say "yes."*
- *If you want to be depressed, I say "yes."*

God said: *I will say yes to any decision you make because that is your free will.* But He also said: *Bear the consequences of your decisions and attitudes because the results will be for every decision made and action taken.* He went further when He told me that an athlete only reaches the level of world competition because he practices and that:

- *Being cheerful is a matter of practice.*
- *Being sad is a matter of practice.*
- *Being good is a matter of practice.*
- *Being happy is a matter of practice.*
- *Being pessimistic is a matter of practice.*
- *Being bad is a matter of practice.*
- *Being optimistic is a matter of practice.*
- *Being an entrepreneur is a matter of practice.*
- *Being depressed is a matter of practice.*
- *Everything you practice will make you good.*

Now that you know, what do you want to practice?

Unfortunately, people today consider their own thoughts but take no steps to improve them. When the mind is not properly educated, it becomes a breeding ground for all kinds of destruction or reckless thoughts, and this almost always results in unproductive and destructive behavior.

People do not care to improve the mind, especially when it comes to health and understanding the body.

The Thought

*Thought is like a powerful weapon. It is
extremely dangerous if it is misused.*
Giles St. Aubyn

David Wallace said:
*"The mind is an excellent servant,
but a cruel master."*

If the person dominates the mind, he is lucky; if he lets himself be dominated by it, he is unhappy. Therefore, a clear and desirable thought to understand the body and serve it is not only to develop all the potential of the mind, but also to avoid the disasters that it can cause to the body. Again, it must be remembered that all the cells in our body work according to the vibrations created by our thoughts. Another thing that we must emphasize is about people who are constantly embarrassed and ashamed of acts they have committed.

Uzma Mazhar, made a dissertation on shame: Shame is the only emotion that attacks the self, making it believe that it is inherently flawed and unpleasant. This crippling emotion destroys self-confidence and prevents you from achieving or enjoying success. When shame enters everyday existence, one is torn between the need to empower and the need to preserve relationships. At that moment, the negative vibrations begin that contribute to cellular deterioration, increases mental damage, and causing mental and physical illnesses.

Educate your thinking, control your emotions, write your goals. Put the power of imagination first, and the path to mental and physical success will be there.

> *"Live in such a way*
> *that if someone speaks badly of you,*
> *nobody will believe it."*

Feeling Sorry For Others

*L*et's talk now about BEING SORRY. People tend to feel sorry for others who go through problems, who are deprived of some organ, who become ill, or who are mentally affected by dementia, or emotional distress caused by the loss of a loved one.

It's normal for this to happen, but it's not good because being sorry is the worst human feeling. Hate can pass, love can end, jealousy can disappear, but pity remains. This feeling is so rooted that it penetrates the smallest details, not only of the body but of the mind whose vibrations will further affect the physical structure.

The ability to see reality is closely linked to the constructive and destructive sectors in times of difficulty. We all know people who suffer from their reasons and cry and say, *how can this be happening to me?* Such people see themselves as victims and live through worship, from the pity that people feel for them. They are extremely creative in providing and building empires of reason to justify their illnesses, not only for others, but mainly for themselves. Some will say: *Yes! ... I think these are really worth it.*

I have seen in patients that the penalty has greatly affected the conditions of the sick, especially the penalty they feel for themselves, which is the worst penalty, the one we feel for ourselves. I see it in patients who have made their illnesses chronic by constantly feeding through the extremely negative penalty. These people are the ones who justify their illnesses by the attitudes of others. They are the people who constantly complain about unattended attention and become in need of affections they will never get.

In the beginning, it is only suffering, until they reach a level of depression that is even worse.

In this book that I titled, *We Are Not What We Eat. We Are What We Do Not Digest and Assimilate*, it is recorded that we should not allow the **ingestion** of negative feelings because they are difficult to digest. When they do not digest, they go into the blood. Serious problem! Everything that is good in the blood dies and is eliminated. Everything that is bad stays and accumulates.

> *Pity penetrates and worsens.*
> *It is the evil that does the most harm.*
> *It is difficult to end it.*

Many people want us to run a hand over their head and say: *Don't worry, you're right.* There are those who are masochists and just like to suffer. There are those who will always find someone to blame. There are those who will always be the victim. There are those who complain about everything. But there are those who really need a word to help them win, to help them move forward. I set myself as an example.

When I was sick, all the doctors I went to told me only

one thing: the cancer has no cure. Each one I consulted, hoping to hear, *"Don't worry; you have a chance,"* actually took away my hope. It was always the same. I wanted to hear something that would uplift my spirit so I could react.

And so, I succumbed, surrendering to the disease, until one day in conversation with God (He speaks to us through thoughts), I asked God: *Why is only 5% of the world's population really successful?* Then he answered me, saying that it was because He helped the 5%. As this penetrated my thoughts, I asked: *Why? Don't you like the other 95%?* And, in response, I understood when I received the message that only the DETERMINED ones are successful. Only the DETERMINED ones receive divine help. It's because that's the divine language!

The doctor I was seeing in the United States decided to put me in "hospice." Hospice is the sector of those who will no longer be medicated. They will only be waiting for death. So I asked him, *"Did you give up on me?"* Without much ceremony, he said that my cancer had no cure and that there was no more medication for my case.

"And my *wishes now, doctor?"* I asked him. He affirmed, and I said: *"I have a wish, and I want my wish to be fulfilled in full."* When he asked me what my wish was, I put forth all the anger, all the indignation in my heart and told him: *"My wish is that you never enter my room again. I'm not going to die lying down. I'm going to die standing up, and I'm still going to bury you one day!"*

That was my moment of DETERMINATION. From then

on, God was showing the ways.

The most interesting thing of all is that every time I felt extremely bad, I tried to stand up, and it got better. Once again, determination was present. I am not a person who lives and feeds the past, but I never saw him again, and I do not even remember his name. But very honestly, I hope he's still alive.

> **Don't let anyone have authority**
> **over your life, over your body.**
> **You have all authority.**

Root Canal Treatment

would like to address root canal treatments. Dentists in California have done a lot of research on root canal treatments.

A tooth, regardless of the material used by the dentist, can accumulate between the bone structure and the tooth, mercury in an amount 3,000 times greater than the body can support. I would like to explain this in a more illustrative way.

Imagine that the mercury in the body, which is normal to exist in a bearable scale, has its transfer through the whole body, passes between the tooth and the bone structure, and communicates with the dental nerve through the pores at the end of the tooth. Since the nerve is not exposed yet, mercury notifies the brain that everything is fine. But if it is not a superficial amount and the nerve is exposed when it passes through the tooth, it receives the communication that the problem is more serious because the nerve is exposed. It notifies the brain, and at this moment, it makes us feel toothache. Now the pain is horrible, and you need to go to the dentist.

The dentist removes the nerve, fills it with any material, and the pain goes away. And now the future problems begin. The mercury that continues its way between the bone structure and the tooth needs to communicate with the nerve. But as the nerve is no longer there, it remains in the same place and accumulates in that area, creating possible infections.

It is very simple for dentists to know if the root canal is causing the accumulation of mercury. When it is necessary to remove a tooth that already has a root canal done, the dentist just needs to remove the tooth horizontally, place the removed tooth horizontally in a glass of water with the necessary transparency to see the tooth. Mercury, a heavy metal accumulated between the outside of the tooth and the inside of the bone structure, will be coming out in the water. It is visible at a glance. As long as there is no discomfort from a possible infection caused by the accumulation of mercury that the body cannot expel, that's fine.

Heavy Metals

Heavy metals, like mercury, are mostly the silent poison that is slowly spreading in the human body. They are present in almost all the foods we consume in our daily lives. In small doses, bearable by the body, they should not cause harm. Notes taken from information on the internet show that current legislation is very strict with the levels of heavy metals in pesticides. Unfortunately, this does not represent greater security for consumers. Many farmers do not use approved pesticides. They buy dangerous products from the black market that have alarming levels of mercury and arsenic. As a consequence, the foods produced with these plants become enriched with these substances. People can spend years overly consuming heavy metals without knowing it. There is still a very serious aggravation. Even after years of using safe pesticides, the soil of these plantations still remains contaminated due to the use of pesticides mainly from illegal ones acquired in the parallel market.

Industry often throws heavy metal waste into the environment without any treatment. This leads to contamination of the entire ecosystem around the factories. Often, these environments also produce food for human consumption, which can lead to population poisoning. Fish are the main concern, as they can contain huge amounts of heavy metals due to bioaccumulation. With each advance in the food chain, the next fish will be more contaminated, since it will have fed on several contaminated organisms thrown into rivers and the sea. The industry, agriculture, and livestock are not concerned with this detail, and the levels of heavy metals in the products we consume as food are becoming alarming.

All of these elements are present in our daily lives, but they need very high concentrations to cause us harm. It is important to know the biological concept about heavy metals that cause negative effects harmful to our health. They are all those that tend to the bioaccumulation process. That is, those that are not metabolized by living organisms and that tend to accumulate, causing diseases. They are reactive because they interact very easily with harmful chemicals, creating physical mutations within our body. (Again, remember that our body was created for transformations, not mutations.) As they are not liable to undergo metabolization, they become a silent enemy that grows and does not allow us to feel the effects on a daily basis, thus damaging the body slowly. This process will lead to the moment when the body will no longer tolerate this enemy and will get sick so that we can take care of it.

These heavy metals are found abundantly in nature and in the inputs used in civil construction and the food industry. Paints for house paintings contained lead, extremely heavy metal, and we were all exposed to this enemy for a long time, creating so-called encephalopathies that create disruptions in the nervous system, in addition to many other physical problems. This relationship was known in the twentieth century, during the autopsy and chemical analysis of the brain of those affected with many diseases of the central nervous system that demonstrated high concentrations of lead. Although health agencies have already warned of this negative effect, the industry, even so, continues to use this metal in the composition of paints. This is because the pharmaceutical industry has not yet determined the relationship between lead and encephalopathy used in the manufacture of paints, especially the toxic metals that contribute too much to feed fungi that, when in excess, cause serious illnesses when they are not expelled and stay in any part of the body.

Although fungi exist as a stage in our body, which undergoes transformations and mutations, when in excess and fermented or inflamed, they can transform healthy cells into cancer cells, especially when the body is in a state of high acidity. Unfortunately, only a few orthomolecular doctors, homeopaths, or therapists suggest a Mineralogram exam to find out if the patient has too much or is deficient in one, where a diet would be required to increase or reduce the quantities found.

But don't worry because these heavy metals[9] can be extracted from the body with some metal extractors, now

9 **EDITOR'S NOTE:** They are called CHELANT substances.

available to those in need. A more specific diet associated with good digestion will bring the body the balance for a healthy life.

At this point, I reserve the right to draw the attention, not only of patients, but also of doctors and therapists, to the need to suggest to patients that they do a mineralogram examination to find out if the patient has too much or is deficient in some metals found in the body. This exam shows all of that. This used to be done by hair testing, but there is now electronic equipment that can detect these anomalies in a few moments.

Evolution moves us away from the nature of normal things to which we always need to be connected. As, for example, considering the initial period of man, there were no bathrooms with toilets, and there was no toilet paper. When I was a child, the financial situation of our family did not allow the use of these items created by the evolution of the times. The bathroom was far from home. It was a hole in the surroundings. There was no toilet. Then it got closer to the house, then it went inside. The vase was already present, then came a simple lid for the vase, then soft and padded lids. At first, it was a bathroom just inside the house. Then there were two. We now have houses with many bathrooms. All this evolution removed us from the reality that the body was not created to defecate sitting, but squatting, where there is the perfect dilation for cleaning through the Colon. The use of toilet paper would not be necessary because the inner part of the anus is put out during the stool extraction period and is collected without the need for the use of toilet paper. Another detail: You do not see an animal stay in the same position at the time of the stool extraction for longer than necessary to defecate.

Toxins From Feces

The bathroom brought into the house and the comfort of the seats created another problem. That is sitting for a long time, forcing the inner part of the anus to remain as if trying to expel the feces that have already left. Many use that time for reading, and now with the creation of the cell phone, a lot of time is spent sitting on the vessel, causing hemorrhoids, which is the non-retraction of the internal part of the anus. Hemorrhoids is also caused by poor digestion of the protein. A kind of glue is accumulated in the blood that makes the red cells stick together. As the body needs to clean itself, it will extract this glue from the blood through the feces, which are stuck to the inner wall of the anus and rectum. In a normal process, when we defecate, residues remain on the inner wall of the anus and rectum, but when we need to defecate again, the old residues come out and the new ones remain. This is the normal process of the body cleaning itself.

When this glue that needs to be expelled comes out in the feces, the residues that should simply be leaning against the inner wall, are glued inside when they should have left. These residues that remain for a long time undergo a fermentation creating a toxin called "acanthocytes" that can go into the bloodstream. They are not feces in the blood. They are toxins due to the fermentation of the feces residues that should have left, but because of the glue, they become trapped creating many diseases mainly in the area where the feces are dispatched. For you to know if your feces come out with glue, when the feces do not fall into the water of the vessel, and it is necessary to give discharges several times for them to come out, it is because surely the feces are coming out with the glue.

For this purpose, the henemas[10] created by the Pharmaceutical industry were developed for internal cleaning of the extracting area. But if there is good digestion, there will be no such glue, the residues would come out normally, and it would not be necessary to clean the area.

10 **REVIEW NOTE:** enteroclysms

Alkaline Body

Now let's talk about alkalinizing the body. Our body needs to remain alkaline so that it can retain oxygen. Oxygen kills cancer cells. The source of life is oxygen. Without it we die almost instantly. We can go for a few days without eating or even without drinking liquid, but without oxygen, it is impossible. And, for that, it is necessary that we can carry oxygen, constantly in our body, through the RBCs (red cells). I remember, once again, that when we inhale oxygen through the mouth or nostrils, and the lung is filled with oxygen, the heart pumps blood to the lung to receive oxygen. It is when the red blood cells, being healthy, receive oxygen on impact against the lung walls and leave carrying oxygen to the body. Twenty-percent of that oxygen goes to the brain. However, for oxygen transport to be complete, through red blood cells (red cells) they must be in order. That is, individually separated, each one of them, without the aggregation caused by the poor digestion of the protein food.

**"This is our job, to breathe and
the heart to pump."**

The proliferation of diseases occurs due to lack of oxygen and several factors originating from poor digestion. The main factors of poor digestion of food are the lack of enzymes initially produced in our body through the mouth. There are two places where more bacteria appear in our body, one is at the entrance (mouth) and the other at the exit. The ones at the entrance, which are the oral enzymes, were placed at the entrance, so they need to enter "alive." Toothpaste kills all of these enzymes necessary for digestion. Poor digestion of food is a deficiency of these enzymes, plus those of our gastric juice. If we make an analysis of the existence of cancer that has existed in the world for a long time, which was openly discovered in 1958, we will have a very important result: toothpaste was introduced massively into the world after the Second World War as of 1946. Poor chewing and without oral enzymes does not carry the oral enzymes necessary for digestion. As cancer can take 5 to 10 years to be detected, only from the years 1955 to 1058 started a great death in the world, and nobody knew why until it was discovered and told to the world that it was a disease called "cancer."

Problems Caused By Fermentation of Feces

Fecal bacteria, as well as feces and toxins that come out, must be removed. At this point, it is also necessary to remember that people eat and exclude food always without problems of constipation, going to the bathroom normally. This, however, does not mean that there was perfect digestion. I had some cancer patients who never had problems with constipation, but, nevertheless, their red blood cells, when analyzing live blood, were shown to be totally grouped, which corresponds to non-digestion of proteins. The foods may have been crushed in the stomach and intestines and never caused problems with defecation. However, the essentials to be digested are proteins, fat, and sugar, which are foods. I did some tests with ozone therapies in some patients, and I could see that there were changes in the blood almost immediately. But the next day, the cells were grouped again. That is, the effect of ozone in the blood is fast, but it is not lasting. The body needs to have its metabolism changed in order to adapt and continue to be well constantly. But a change in metabolism does not occur overnight.

They were anomalies acquired in the course of life, and they do not come out immediately. We can even get momentary cures, but illnesses tend to return. This is the case of cancer. Most people, after medical treatments, suffer recession, the cancer coming back. It is not an apparent cure that will bring tranquility to the patient. The most important thing is that the body no longer gets sick. With clean blood, there is no disease left in the body.

Another Warning

A few years after I gave a course on Morphology of the Living Blood in Aracajú (Brazil) going to Rio de Janeiro where my wife was waiting for me. When I sat down in the plane, I felt an intense pain in my chest and almost could not breathe. I immediately thought that it could not be happening to me, having a stroke, having a heart attack, because my blood was clean, and that I was sure of.

Right after takeoff, I went to the bathroom, sat down on the toilet, took off my shirt, put wet paper on my head, and started doing breathing techniques to see if the pain would stop. I stood still for a long time waiting for the pain to improve. It improved, but it wasn't completely gone. I didn't even want to move my arms because when I moved, the pain intensified.

When I arrived at the nonstop landing that was in Brasilia, where I should change planes, I called my wife, told her what was happening, and asked her to get a cardiologist right away. As soon as I arrived, we went to the doctor who did all my cardiologic exams and found no abnormalities in my heart.

He then called another doctor to check on me. The

same thing. He did not find anything to justify the pain I was feeling. The last doctor to examine me suggested that I do an ultrasound scan and referred me to an ultrasound school where her friend was teaching at the time. When we got there, I immediately went to the room where the devices were. I sat on a bed, and the teacher with her students behind her started the ultrasound process. She pointed the pistol at different parts of my body, such as the shoulder, arm, neck, but did not point at my chest where I felt the pain. So, I took the teacher's hand and pointed the machine at my chest where I felt the pain. I said to her, "This is it, doctor, where I feel the pain." She very calmly asked the students where they saw what was causing my chest pain. They all said it was on the left shoulder. She pointed out to me the place on my left shoulder where the pain originated, which reflected in the chest looking like a heart attack. She reassured me, saying that I should be calm because my heart had nothing wrong. If I had gone to a doctor who did not understand this kind of problem, I would already hace been asked for heart surgery.

At that moment, I remembered that when I arrived in the city where I was going to teach the days before, when I was taking the microscope case from the trunk, a very hurried lady had pushed me wanting to get off the plane, and the suitcase almost fell. I took the suitcase, which was heavy, with my left arm so it wouldn't fall, and I felt a slight discomfort in my left shoulder. I told the ultrasound teacher this fact, and she without hesitation confirmed that it was possibly because of this that there was a slight anomaly in the shoulder nerves causing that chest pain.

Here is my recommendation to anyone who could see what I felt in my chest: do an ultrasound scan before any operative decision.

Free Radicals

What are free radicals, and what do they cause in the human body?

The Brunswick Biomedical Technologies Laboratory, which tested numerous formulations, describes the effects of free radical damage:

In general, free radicals cause the development of at least 50 diseases! A partial list includes arthritis and other inflammatory diseases, kidney disease, cataracts, inflammatory bowel disease, colitis, lung dysfunction, pancreatitis, drug reactions, skin lesions, and aging, to name a few. Heart disease and cancer are two of the most common diseases associated with free radical damage. Heart disease is the leading cause of death in the United States today, killing about one in three Americans. Literally, free radicals are the main factor in aging. Soon, the heart acquires premature aging properties.

Other disease states for which free radicals are responsible are Parkinson's disease, Alzheimer's disease, lupus, atherosclerosis, strokes, rheumatoid arthritis, age-related hearing loss, liver disease, age-related neurological disorders, retinopathy, muscle degeneration, symptoms of TMJ, and cerebral palsy, Down syndrome, ALS, sepsis, Huntington's disease, loss of skin elasticity (collagen collapse), and the list is still growing as the research continues. There are more than 300 theories to explain the phenomenon of aging. Among all theories, the free radical theory of aging, first proposed by Dr. Denham Harman at the University of Nebraska, is the most accepted, popular, and widely tested. Aging is believed to occur as a result of constant exposure to reactive oxygen species from free radicals with cumulative damage over a lifetime, along with gradually decreasing repair capacity and increasing degenerative changes in individual organs, tissues, and cells. The body has enzymes that can repair many of the damaged proteins, but when those enzymes are damaged, the repair processes are compromised.

"Nowadays, it is difficult to open any medical journal and not find any article about the role of 'Reactive Oxygen Species' or 'free radicals' in human disease." The species have been implicated in more than 50 diseases. This large number suggests that radicals are not something esoteric, but that they participate as a fundamental component of tissue damage in most, if not all, human diseases."

American Journal of Medicine article, 9/30/1991 v91 n3C p12S (9); Oxidants and Antioxidants: Pathophysiological Determinants and Therapeutic Agents, Author: Halliwell, Barry.

There are many internal and external factors that form free radicals: tobacco smoke, excess alcohol, radiation including ultraviolet radiation from the sun, car exhaust, pesticides, herbicides, pollution, use of prescription drugs, chemotherapy, surgery, breakdown of bacteria by white blood cells, microbial or viral infections, toxin metabolism, inflammatory processes, by-products of oxygen metabolism, stress, shock, trauma, hypoxia, enzymatic reactions, calorie consumption, poor diet, and many food materials, especially the oxidation of hydrogenated oils. A single free radical can destroy an enzyme, a protein molecule, a DNA strand or an entire cell, but even worse, in a single second it can trigger torrential chain reactions in our body. Each free radical can initiate and perpetuate millions of other free radicals, triggering chains of biologically damaging reactions. This damage is at the molecular and cellular levels. Ironically, the underlying mechanism that most chemotherapeutic agents and ionizing radiation have is not to neutralize free radicals, but to produce more free radicals that lead to irreversible tissue damage. Free radicals are not visible in the blood, but we can see during the analysis of living blood, the damage caused by them.

"Mens sana in corpore sano corpore sano"
"Clean mind, clean body."

This was the "Great Response" of Juvenal, the Roman thinker, poet, and philosopher, about which a human being should want more in their life: Clean mind, or clean body? The emotions we experience are in constant vibration, creating, transforming, or mutating what exists in our body. Our thoughts are like radio waves, always on the same frequency. And they are transmitted every second to the entire universe and mainly to our body, which receives more quickly because it is the closest. People always blame their illnesses for circumstances and forget what circumstances we create.

Everything in the Universe is vibrating. Because we are carbon, and matter was created through energy via energy, although undergoing changes, will continue to operate the transformations continually. Conny Méndez, in his *"Four in One Metaphysics,"* states that as we see created things—man, plants, flowers, earth, water, insects, animals, birds, and fish, we know they exist because they vibrate. Our brain that receives, stores and makes its communications, will always be sending the results of these vibrations that we create to our body. Decisions for a healthy life are like seeds that are planted. They require that they be cared for and watered daily for them to grow. If you say you made the decision and do nothing to make it happen, you will never reach your goal. We get sick long before the disease appears. This is because we do not obey our body's needs and demands.

We do not maintain the body. We do not create prevention. In short, we allow the disease to proliferate until the moment comes when the body cannot take it anymore and shows the symptoms. It is because we are doing everything wrong. In order to better understand the concept that *we are not what we eat; we are what we do not digest*, we need to know that any food from our planet—land or sea—has the three basic foods for the survival of the living being.

Protein • Fat • Sugar
Our job is just one! "Digest the three."

***We are not what we eat; we are
what we digest and assimilate.***

If you are digesting, you can eat poison that does not die, and it will come out in the feces, in the urine, in the sweat. It will come out somehow.

However, if you don't digest, it goes to the blood. That is a very big problem because everything that is good and needed in the blood then dies, while everything that is bad is taking over and accumulating.

***If we don't have time to take care of
our health now, we will have to find time
to take care of illness later.***

When Squeezed

*L*ook at the results of thoughts and attitudes. Solomon once said, "We are what we think." There is no doubt about that statement.

Let's compare some of the natural laws of all the elements in the universe. If we squeeze an orange, orange juice will come out, never mango. If we squeeze a mango, passion fruit juice will certainly not come out. From those who have hatred within them, surely hatred will emerge. From those who have sadness inside, sadness will emerge. From those who store joy, joy will be what we see. From the one who has the spirit of defeat within, defeat and failure will emerge. From the one who has the spirit of victory within him, it will be a victor that we will see. And surely, from the one who has love, love will come out as divine essence.

And now, if we could squeeze you who are reading this closing statement, what would come out? What kind of result would we find? Have you already made this assessment for yourself, or have you not yet discovered what is inside of you?

Reflections
By Jimmy Albuquerque

There are absolute laws governing happiness. You have Divine strength keeping you and your health in order, and in total universal harmony. That strength that is within you, where knowledge is stored, does not speak … but listen carefully … if you call, it comes through the decision!

The Universe is governed by natural laws, and everything starts with dreams and hope. We all dream. Some dream of almost nothing, and others of much. In reality, we are the size of our thoughts because we are what we think we are. God created men alike, with the right to search the mental reserve of the Universe for all the resources necessary for mental and spiritual development. We are spiritual beings and have the right to use these reserves created and left by God. You and I are all part of a single Universal mind. We are individual expressions of a Universal mind and of all the force of Nature, where all the knowledge exists and will come to exist. And, if God has given us this ability, we must always remember that the world is in the hands of those who have the ability to dream and run the risk of living their dreams.

—Jimmy Albuquerque

For you who have finished reading
this book, may happiness and love
be an integral part of your life.

About The Author

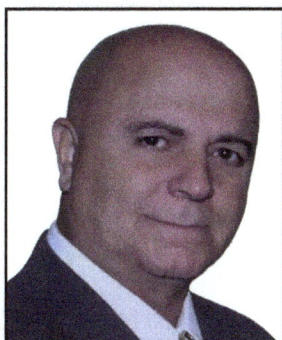

Jimmy Albuquerque

JIMMY ALBUQUERQUE's birth name and at his baptism was Jurandir Teixeira de Albuquerque.

Today, he occupies a leading positioned place in the world as a Seminarian, Morphologist (analysis of live blood), Micro-biologist, Clinic Naturapy Doctor's degree, and bio-doctor's degree. He has lectured in different countries, such as Italy, England, Germany, Belgium, Mexico, Colombia, Brazil, and the United States, where he has lived for over 50 years. After his recovery from a considered uncurable cancer in his brain (GBM-grade 4 cancer), he improved his knowledge in various areas concerning mental health and physics, adding values that complete his work as morphologist. Besides being a Notary in the United States, he became a master coach, a coach to better identify the problems of his patients.

Jimmy graduated from courses like Emotional Intelligence, Iridology, and Reiki. He was president of Fenate (National Federation of Therapists) and was actually Marshal for Human Rights in Brazil. He received in the United States the

Immigrant Trophy of the Year in 2009, and Hero of the Brazilian Community by the International Brazilian Press in 2018.

On October 3, 2019, he received the Personality of the Year award by the *London Fame* magazine.

***

After his recovery, Jimmy developed his therapy to help his own family remain healthy and not get sick.

Today, he uses this therapy to help many people, to contribute to cures, and to prevent various diseases, including cancer, working with the aspects of physical, mental, and spiritual work for better results.

The initial therapy for all patients is to receive "the little hug." After the visit, they part with "the big hug."

Contact:
E-mail: bloodanalysis@live.com
Instagram: @jimmyalbuquerque
YouTube: Jimmy Albuquerque
Facebook: jimmyalbuquerque.5
Telephone: 754-232-2068

A book
that is at odds
with everything
we've learned.

www.ingramcontent.com/pod-product-compliance
Lightning Source LLC
Chambersburg PA
CBHW040143270326
41928CB00023B/3334